LIVING PARKINSON'S

PRAISE FOR LIVING PARKINSON'S

"Movement is medicine, and community is power. *Living Parkinson's* brings both to life—showing how exercise, optimism and connection can help anyone with Parkinson's find joy and strength in each day."

DAVIS PHINNEY, Olympian, and Founder of the Davis Phinney Foundation

"Steve Yellen understands something fundamental about living with Parkinson's: Everyone needs a plan. In *Living Parkinson's*, he lays out seven practical, inspiring strategies—attitude, knowledge, support, exercise, wellness, advocacy and research—and shows how putting them into daily action can transform fear into purpose and transition uncertainty into agency. This book is a roadmap for reclaiming control, staying engaged and living a full life. It is a powerful reminder that we are not defined by Parkinson's; however, we can be defined by how we rise to meet it."

MICHAEL S. OKUN, MD, co-author of *The New York Times* best seller,
The Parkinson's Plan

"People like Steve Yellen who are directly affected by Parkinson's disease will change the course of it for all of us. In *Living Parkinson's*, Steve gives you a guided tour of living the best life you can with this disease, which we should work to end."

RAY DORSEY, MD, co-author of *The Parkinson's Plan*

"*Living Parkinson's* is required reading for anyone who's been diagnosed with the disease. It's divided into easy-to-digest sections that don't overwhelm, and ultimately the reader comes away with a doable action plan. As someone who has had the disease for six years now, I found it incredibly inspiring, and no doubt care partners will come away with a deeper understanding of what their loved one is going through. Uplifting, hopeful and well-researched."

FIONA DAVIS, *NY Times* bestselling author and
member of the Michael J. Fox Patient Council

"This is the book I wish had been out when I was first diagnosed. It contains so many wise nuggets that it has taken me years to accumulate. An essential guide to taking on Parkinson's from every angle."

CATHY MOLOHAN, Board Member of Parkinson's Europe,
Ambassador, World Parkinson's Congress

"Research and experience both show that people can live fulfilling lives with Parkinson's disease. Fulfillment often depends on how one approaches the condition. Those who maintain a positive *Attitude*, seek *Knowledge* about their disease and ways to manage it, build a strong team for *Support*, show the *Fight* to overcome challenges and pursue *Wellness*, engage in *Advocacy* for themselves and others and appreciate how *Research* can shape their future are most likely to live well with Parkinson's. Steve's book presents these "Seven Pillars of Wisdom" in a clear, practical and inspiring way."

DR. DANIEL M. CORCOS, Professor of Physical Therapy and
Human Movement Sciences, Northwestern University

"From diagnosis through team-building, community, wellness and advocacy, this is your go-to guide. Keep it close and open the chapter that fits the moment. With personal stories and truly actionable advice, it's practical, hopeful and grounded."

LARRY GIFFORD, President and Co-Founder, PD Avengers

"No one likes to be alone on a journey, especially if it's a difficult one, and with this book, author Steve Yellen has created an authentic, practical and inspiring companion for anyone on a Parkinson's journey. *Living Parkinson's* blends evidence-informed guidance, personal insight and actionable tools into a worthy addition to every Parkinson's bookshelf!"

ANDRÉA MERRIAM, CEO, Parkinson & Movement Disorder Alliance

"Steve has written an informative and engaging book that provides people with Parkinson's disease the tools and strategies needed to support and sustain long-term engagement in physical activity. This approach is so important because a big limitation in Parkinson's disease management is that people often don't stay engaged with exercise, sometimes starting strong but then dropping off. The book aligns with my research focused on physical activity interventions by helping individuals build the confidence, knowledge and greater sense of control necessary to apply strategies and build habits that last in their daily lives."

DR. LORI QUINN, Director of the Neurorehabilitation Research Lab
at Teachers College at Columbia University

"*Living Parkinson's* is Steve Yellen's roadmap to slowing down the progression of Parkinson's disease. He is an inspirational role model who has spelled out all the steps he takes to live well with Parkinson's. I highly recommend his book that helps connect the dots to spark the warrior within all of us who are faced with the challenge of fighting this disease."

MARGIE ALLEY, 2026 World Parkinson's Congress Ambassador
PingPongParkinson World Championships medalist

"Steve's book is a powerful guide to empowerment. Thoughtfully written, it offers practical advice for individuals with Parkinson's, encouraging them to take control of their condition in every way they can. The book emphasizes two key strategies: gaining a deep understanding of Parkinson's and its treatments and staying physically active for as long as possible. For those facing the challenges of Parkinson's, this book provides valuable insights that can help make the journey more manageable and hopeful."

DR. ROY ALCALAY, Chief of the Movement Disorders Division at
Tel Aviv Sourasky Medical Center, Israel

"All too often, Parkinson's disease gets mistaken for an 'old man's disease' when in reality, it does not discriminate based on race, age or gender. As a member of the Young Onset Parkinson's Disease (YOPD) community for the last 18 years and counting, it's refreshing to see a book written *by* a person with YOPD that can serve as a guide *for* others diagnosed with YOPD to live their best life!"

ANNA GRILL, Founder of the Young Onset Parkinson's Network,
a program of the PMD Alliance

"Steve Yellen celebrates the spirit of living with Parkinson's: the joy in movement, the power of connection and the unwavering belief that every person can thrive. His words shine a light on what is possible, and that sense of possibility is the heartbeat of our community. What he offers here is nothing short of encouragement in motion."

LYNN HAGERBRANT, Co-Founder, Parkinson's Body & Mind,
Co-Chair, Michael J. Fox Foundation Patient Council

"Insightful and immediately useful, *Living Parkinson's* meets people where they are and helps them take the next step—whether through exercise, mindful routines or community engagement. Its whole-person approach reflects evidence-based strategies and shared stories that can support wellness in all facets of life."

Brian Grant Foundation

"Steve Yellen's personal story and insights provide invaluable guidance for the Parkinson's community in promoting a proactive approach to living with the disease. In *Living Parkinson's*, Steve emphasizes the importance of exercise and movement and underscores our belief that physical activity can significantly enhance the quality of life for those living with Parkinson's."

STEVE ANNEAR, Chief Executive Officer,
The Kirk Gibson Foundation for Parkinson's

"Every Parkinson's journey is different. But Steve Yellen's guide reminds us that the journey doesn't need to be taken alone. There's a global community out there to learn from, lean on and find inspiration to take control. *Living Parkinson's* is incredibly practical, easy to navigate and told with warmth and humour. A vital guide for everyone with Parkinson's, wherever you are in the world."

CAROLINE RASSELL, CEO, Parkinson's UK

"Steve's *Living Parkinson's* is a practical guide to finding freedom within Parkinson's—not freedom from the diagnosis, but freedom through movement, connection, knowledge and everyday choices. His book is divided into simple, accessible sections that make it easy to absorb without feeling overwhelmed. Whether you're newly diagnosed or years into the journey, you walk away with a foundation to develop your own plan and a stronger sense of what living well can look like. It's honest, hopeful and grounded in real experience. A powerful, easy read that seeks to leave you better equipped and more prepared to live well with Parkinson's."

EMMA COLLIN, CEO, Fight Parkinson's (Australia)

"*Living Parkinson's* is a call to reclaim the story. It reminds us that Parkinson's may change the path, but it does not define the life—purpose, movement and community do. Written from lived experience, this guide empowers people to take control, keep moving forward and surround themselves with the support they need to not just endure, but to truly thrive."

SCOTT TOWNSEND, Vice-President, Philanthropy, Brand Marketing & Communications, Parkinson Canada

LIVING PARKINSON'S

7 Strategies for Living a Full Life with Renewed Purpose

STEVE YELLEN

Living Parkinson's

First paperback edition February 2026

Cover photo by Olivia Przop

ISBN 979-8-218-88347-8 (paperback)

Published by Living Parkinson's Press

www.livingparkinsons.com

Disclaimer

TABLE OF CONTENTS

PREFACE

There are many books on Parkinson's written by doctors and researchers covering its history, causes, symptoms and medical treatments. This isn't one of them. *Living Parkinson's* is about taking charge of your personal journey and facing the future with positivity and purpose.

You've probably heard the phrase, "No two people with Parkinson's are the same." It's true! Parkinson's is often called a "snowflake disease" because it affects everyone uniquely. But beyond Parkinson's itself, each of us is wired differently, with our own strengths, limitations and motivations. That's why no single path works for everyone. What I can offer is the approach that works for me and that I hope can inspire you.

This book offers seven empowering strategies that are helping me fight back—and that anyone can use as a roadmap to overcome challenges, celebrate wins and stay focused on their personal fight:

- ▶ **ATTITUDE:** Prepare to win your battle
- ▶ **KNOWLEDGE:** Take control through learning
- ▶ **SUPPORT:** Build and strengthen your team
- ▶ **FIGHT:** Make exercise your medicine
- ▶ **WELLNESS:** Be your best self
- ▶ **ADVOCACY:** Make your voice heard
- ▶ **RESEARCH:** Help advance the science

Living Parkinson's isn't a one-size-fits-all approach—it's a guide filled with personal stories, insights from experts in the field and practical tools you can adapt to build your own plan. It's written by someone living that journey every day, striving to live his best life *and* contribute to the fight for all of us.

Each chapter focuses on a strategy and includes:

▶ What you'll learn

▶ My personal experiences that you can adapt to your own journey

▶ Research, practical tips and real examples

▶ Insights from top experts

▶ Stories of others *Living Parkinson's*

▶ "What You Can Do" callouts

▶ A space to capture your takeaways and action plans

I wrote this book with the idea that every reader can take something away from it—something that will improve their own journey. But I need to say up front: Please don't feel like you have to do exactly what I do.

At the time I'm writing *Living Parkinson's*, it's been more than six years since my diagnosis. The plan I've built for myself has taken that long to develop—through plenty of trial and error. Some things have worked really well, and others just weren't right for me (I'll share a few examples along the way).

With each of the strategies in this book, I started small and gradually built on what worked as I became more comfortable and learned what was realistic for me. You'll see plenty of examples of routines and goals that have become part of my daily life—but that doesn't mean they need to become part of yours.

Think of this book as a menu, not a checklist. It offers options you can try, adapt or skip altogether. You may even find other approaches that fit within these strategies—or some that fall completely outside of them—that work for you. If you start by choosing just one or two things that resonate with you, like shifting your mindset, learning more about your condition, joining a group or simply adding one extra exercise to your routine, then you're moving in the right direction. Progress begins with small, consistent steps, not by doing everything at once.

In short, there's no single prescription that works for everyone, and there shouldn't be. As you'll hear me say throughout this book, everyone is on their *own* path and needs to build their *own* plan. My goal is simply to inspire you to find the formula that's right for you and to use it to live your best possible life. That is *Living Parkinson's*.

COMPANION WEBSITE: Additional resources and updates are available on my website at livingparkinsons.com. There, you can also subscribe to the *Living Parkinson's* newsletter.

MY PLEDGE: A portion of any proceeds from *Living Parkinson's* will be donated to research, community and philanthropic organizations working to improve the lives of people with the disease.

*"The greatest discovery of my generation
is that human beings can alter their lives
by altering their attitudes of mind."*

WILLIAM JAMES

Start Your Journey Strong

Getting a Parkinson's diagnosis is a gut punch. I imagine everyone remembers the moment they were told they have this incurable neurodegenerative disease. But that's where the commonality ends. Both before and after diagnosis, each person's journey is deeply personal and unique.

Some people I've met felt a strange sense of relief when they finally got their diagnosis after years of unexplained symptoms, frustrating misdiagnoses or painful and ineffective procedures. For me, it was the opposite. I was in good health, aside from a minor tremor. I expected my appointment with a neurologist to be routine and to walk away with a simple diagnosis. Then—*BAM!* Out of nowhere, I was told I had Parkinson's. It was life-changing.

What follows the diagnosis is just as individual as the moment itself. For me, it began with a long period of quiet denial. I accepted the diagnosis in words, but not yet in actions. Over time, that changed. As I learned more, I became more proactive. Eventually, I took full control of my plan and began managing my Parkinson's aggressively on my terms.

It's important to recognize that while getting past denial and reaching genuine acceptance is a very personal process, it's nonetheless a crucial step. This may sound blunt, but the longer you stay in denial, the longer you delay your ability to move forward. And moving forward with resilience and positivity is the goal behind *Living Parkinson's*.

CHAPTER 1

ATTITUDE

Prepare to Win Your Battle

Ownership is everything. The moment you take control, your fight begins.

WHAT YOU'LL LEARN IN THIS CHAPTER

▶ Why attitude is your first and most important tool

▶ The specific attitude that can lead to better overall disease management and quality of life

▶ How one psychological concept—self-efficacy—can be the spark that changes everything

▶ The steps you can take to build resilience and self-efficacy

▶ How to define your personal objective and use it to guide your plan

Living Parkinson's is an attitude. I can't tell you how many times I have heard people say, "Don't let Parkinson's define you." I disagree. *Living Parkinson's* is about acknowledging my Parkinson's and not turning away. Looking it straight in the eyes and focusing on it every day. Using it as motivation to accomplish what I've set my mind to do that day to keep the disease at bay.

I embrace the challenge and have made it my life's purpose to beat this disease. It's my reason for getting out of bed in the morning—*not* my excuse for avoiding the day—and it's embodied in the hashtag I often use: #NeverGiveUp.

To commemorate this "relationship" with Parkinson's, I had the Parkinson's tulip tattooed on my shoulder. This tulip is the internationally recognized symbol for Parkinson's disease awareness.

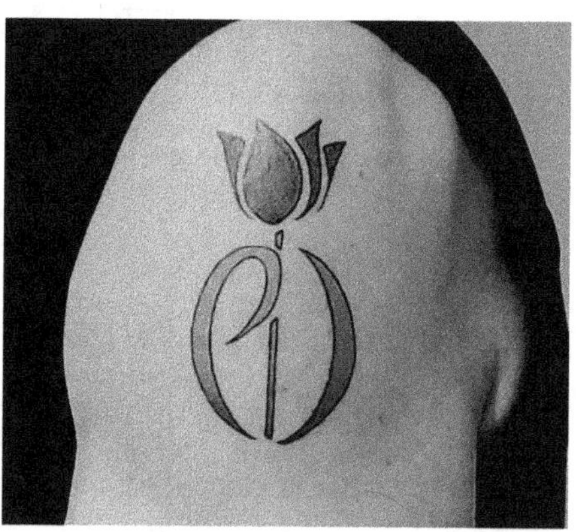

My Parkinson's Tulip Tattoo

I've met a lot of people with Parkinson's since my diagnosis. What I've seen firsthand is that those who confront the disease head-on and have an attitude of "Tell me everything I can do to battle this" do better at managing their journey.

THE DIAGNOSIS THAT CHANGED EVERYTHING

On July 17, 2019, I walked into the neurologist's office as a healthy, fit 55-year-old with a slight tremor in my left hand. I was eager to get an idea of what was causing it and get to work. Instead, after an examination that included a series of finger taps, hand flips and foot stamps, the doctor left the room and returned with a sentence that would change my life:

"You have Parkinson's disease."

A few months earlier, when my wife had ironically half-joked that the tremor might be Parkinson's, we had both laughed it off. Now, hearing those words out loud, I was stunned. Still, I did what I always do: I went to work. I compartmentalized the news, called my wife from the car to tell her and carried on with my day.

The neurologist told me that Parkinson's does not significantly reduce your lifespan. But it wasn't until days later that I had the courage to google "Parkinson's disease life expectancy." I wasn't ready to face what I might find.

I clung to the hope that the diagnosis was a mistake. Could I *really* have Parkinson's? I sought additional opinions—first at Mount Sinai because I'd heard they had treated Michael J. Fox, then at Yale. But each time, the answer was the same: I had Parkinson's. One doctor even told me there was "nothing special" about my case—I just had Parkinson's. Really? *Just* Parkinson's?!?!

They all offered the same comforting message: Parkinson's wouldn't significantly reduce my lifespan. In hindsight, I think that phrase stuck with me more than anything else. It minimized the threat. It enabled me to rationalize, to wait and to change nothing.

LIVING LIKE NOTHING CHANGED

In the year following my diagnosis, I didn't change my lifestyle, my diet or my approach to address the disease. I went on living almost as if I hadn't been diagnosed at all.

In early 2021, I participated in the PD GENEration genetic study and learned that I didn't have any of the genes linked to

Parkinson's. I wondered what else could have caused it. During the 1980s, I had been exposed to trichloroethylene[1] (TCE) both at a summer job in a commercial print shop and during graduate school in a semiconductor lab. I had also suffered a head injury in a car accident in 1987. Both, I later learned, could have contributed, but I will never know for sure.

Because I hadn't noticed any progression of my symptoms in those first two years, I allowed myself to believe that this slight tremor was everything Parkinson's had in store for me, or that it would progress so slowly I would never have to face up to its realities. This lulled me into a passive, hands-off approach when it came to doing anything differently, and I didn't change anything in my daily routine.

I'm really not sure why, as I've always prided myself on dealing with challenges head-on. Maybe it was the magnitude of the diagnosis or the lack of noticeable changes in my symptoms, but I was more than happy to bury my head in the sand and stay there.

MOMENT ONE: THE WAKE-UP CALL

That all changed when I went in for my next exam with my movement disorder specialist, at which point I learned that my Unified Parkinson's Disease Rating Scale (UPDRS) score had increased. The UPDRS is a rating tool used to gauge the severity and progression of Parkinson's disease in patients. The results shattered my illusion that I was a special case, immune to progression. Based on the results, my doctor recommended I start on Sinemet® (levodopa/carbidopa), which I would have to take for the rest of my life.

The finality of that prescription was a major setback. I'd always enjoyed good health and viewed any medication—especially a long-term prescription—as something of a defeat. And now here I was, facing a lifelong course of medicine and the realization that, in no uncertain terms, Parkinson's was gaining ground on me.

Sometimes, though, the best things come from moments like that. From that instant—*Moment One*—I decided I was going to be in control. I had a new purpose in life: to do everything possible in my power to beat this disease.

What You Can Do: Claim Your Moment One

Even if you haven't been proactive in your Parkinson's journey, you can still flip the switch yourself and take back control. How? Decide that today is your Moment One.

Another important milestone in my journey was taking part in the Pre-Active PD study at Columbia University in 2022. This study looked at how working with an occupational therapist impacts a person's motivation and activity levels. In this study, I was assigned an occupational therapist (as opposed to the control group, which was not). I learned a great deal more about exercise and its benefits in battling Parkinson's (more on exercise in Chapter 4 and on research studies in Chapter 7).

Over a three-month period, I had five informative sessions with an occupational therapist. I learned that my exercise routine needed to contain aerobic, resistance, balance and flexibility components; that I needed to exercise for 150 minutes per week; and that using an activity watch would enable me to track my progress.

I immediately went out and bought a Fitbit® watch so I could measure my activity. I felt lucky to have been in the group that was assigned a therapist—I now had a weapon in my battle with Parkinson's. What I learned in the Pre-Active PD study played a key role in accelerating my efforts to take charge of my condition and ignite the journey that had begun at Moment One.

MOMENT TWO: THE WEAPON I NEEDED

By 2023, I was motivated in my fight to beat the disease. I was exercising vigorously based on what I had learned in the Pre-Active PD study, and engaged in the local Parkinson's community. Little did I know that another key moment was coming at the CT Parkinson's Symposium on March 24, 2023. I had just seen a presentation by Dr. Sule Tinaz of Yale University on a small proof-of-concept study that showed high-intensity aerobic exercise preserved dopamine-producing neurons, the brain cells that are most vulnerable to destruction in patients with Parkinson's.

She showed a slide with two brain scans, one taken before the study began and one taken after the same person had spent six months exercising at a high intensity. The after-scan brain was lit up, clearly showing a stronger dopamine signal. Here was proof I could see with my own eyes that there might be a way for me to take control of my Parkinson's! Exercise was the answer.

After her presentation, Dr. Tinaz didn't get many questions and the mood in the room didn't change. I was shocked—I had expected there would be a line of people waiting to speak to her to learn more about what they could do for themselves, but I was the only person standing there.

I told Dr. Tinaz how excited I was to hear about her results and also how surprised I was that the audience reaction was so muted. "This is fantastic!" I said. "I've been looking for something I could do to take control of my Parkinson's. I can't wait to get started!"

"That attitude is a great example of self-efficacy," she told me.

Self-*what*? I had never heard the term before. But I immediately grasped the concept given I had experienced it before. It changed everything! This time, I couldn't wait to get home and google "self-efficacy." I seized upon Dr. Tinaz's research and started on my quest to build an exercise program that could put a halt to my Parkinson's progression. But as I learned more about self-efficacy, my focus shifted from the research itself to something just as life-changing.

That was Moment Two, when I was handed the weapon that could give me the edge I needed to win my battle with Parkinson's: self-efficacy.

What You Can Do: Shift Your Attitude

It doesn't matter whether you were diagnosed last week, last year or ten years ago—you *can* change your attitude and reframe your personal battle with Parkinson's. I hope that *Living Parkinson's* can be a factor in sparking a change of attitude for you. If it does, it will have served its purpose.

WHAT IS SELF-EFFICACY?

So, what did my Google search for self-efficacy tell me? Self-efficacy is a term coined by psychologist Albert Bandura referring to a belief in one's ability to succeed in specific situations or to accomplish a task. People with high self-efficacy are more motivated, persistent and resilient—even when faced with challenges.

Individuals with high self-efficacy are more likely to engage in challenging tasks, persist in the face of adversity and quickly recover from setbacks. Another way to think about self-efficacy is having the attitude of facing challenges with the belief that you can control your destiny. Adopting a goal-oriented approach that yields a series of small, progressive wins serves as proof of your ability to succeed at the larger effort.

Why was I so intrigued by this? Self-efficacy had always played a big role in my life (even though I hadn't known what it was called), and I knew it could particularly help me in this new battle with Parkinson's. Self-efficacy was and is a core part of my attitude, and if I could build on it and use it to my advantage, it could play a key role in helping me beat Parkinson's. I thought about how I had responded to setbacks (primarily injuries) in the past, and saw a pattern.

In 1987, I was in a car accident. Hit by a drunk driver, I suffered a head injury and was in the hospital for a few days. I remember asking my parents to bring my dumbbells so I could keep exercising while I was recovering. A little extreme, I know, but possibly a manifestation of my self-efficacy. Just doing *something* while being bedridden in the hospital made me feel more in control and represented a return to normal life.

Individuals with high self-efficacy are more likely to engage in challenging tasks, persist in the face of adversity and quickly recover from setbacks.

In 2007, I had knee surgery. My physical therapist prescribed ankle mobility exercises three days a week. I remember asking him, "If three days a week is good, can I do them seven days a week?" Of course, I did.

As I compare these examples and others in my professional life to the passive attitude I'd had before Moment One, I feel almost embarrassed—it's as if I had missed an opportunity for a few years after my diagnosis. How could I have been so passive in my reaction to being diagnosed? Was it the doctors telling me that the disease doesn't seriously impact life expectancy? Was it that I hadn't noticed the worsening of my symptoms? I don't know, but ever since Moment Two, I've worked my hardest to make up for lost time by doing even more. It's been life-changing for me.

I had come to understand something that was core to my personality. Since self-efficacy is a defined psychological concept, I could learn about ways to nurture it and enhance it. To take control of my fight to beat Parkinson's, I needed to learn as much as I could about the journey I was on and build a plan of attack—and not let up.

I focused more on exercise-driven goals, and I finished my first Spartan® race in Boston with my son Zack on November 12, 2022, two days after my 59th birthday. That was the start of my renewed passion for athletic events, spurred on by the goal-oriented aspect of self-efficacy. I started taking a more proactive role in my treatment, constantly looking for other options (supplements, Eastern medicines, etc.) that might slow my progression. And I began reaching out to other Parkinson's warriors I found online to share stories, giving me confidence that I was on the right path.

Self-efficacy has played a crucial role for me, and it can likewise play one for you in managing your Parkinson's (or other life challenges). It provides the motivation needed to maintain a positive attitude, stick to treatments and impact overall health outcomes. It's a concept that people living with Parkinson's are increasingly using to take a more proactive role in managing their condition. And isn't taking control of this disease exactly what we all want?

Self-efficacy has empowered me to build both resilience and optimism as I go through my journey, enabling me to better manage the symptoms and progression. I believe it can do the same for you, too, and become the spark to get you started *Living Parkinson's*.

SELF-EFFICACY
The Psychological Concept

In his paper introducing the concept, "Self-Efficacy: Toward a Unifying Theory of Behavioral Change,"[2,3] Albert Bandura identifies four primary sources that shape self-efficacy (each aligns with the strategies outlined in this book):

MASTERY EXPERIENCES: Personal successes reinforce an individual's belief in their abilities. A goal-setting approach is integral to self-efficacy as it influences motivation, effort and perseverance. In health contexts, successfully managing symptoms or adhering to a treatment plan can increase confidence in one's ability to maintain their well-being.[4]

VICARIOUS EXPERIENCES: Observing others successfully complete a task can strengthen one's own belief in their capabilities. It provides the confidence that achieving similar success is indeed attainable.

VERBAL PERSUASION: Encouragement from others can enhance self-efficacy. Healthcare providers, family and support groups play a vital role in reinforcing positive beliefs about health management.[5]

PHYSIOLOGICAL AND EMOTIONAL STATES: Positive emotions and physical well-being can boost self-efficacy, while stress and anxiety can negatively impact it. Being in the right state of mind will increase the chances for success.

Research has shown that Parkinson's patients with higher self-efficacy scores had better motor and non-motor symptomatology and quality of life.[6]

HOW THE RIGHT ATTITUDE HELPS IN BATTLING PARKINSON'S

Your attitude can be a powerful ally in managing your Parkinson's journey. Research (by Bandura) has shown that people with a high degree of self-efficacy who take a proactive approach fare better in dealing with health issues and experience a better quality of life. For me, cultivating this sense of empowerment has been transformative. Here's how self-efficacy has shaped my own experience and how it can benefit you in your battle:

PROACTIVELY MANAGE YOUR CONDITION: This means continuously exploring new avenues, whether those are specific exercises, beneficial supplements or alternative (Eastern-based) approaches—all aimed at slowing the progression of the disease. The steps I've taken have helped me manage the disease in the best possible way, enabling me to maintain the high quality of life I've enjoyed to this point.

ADHERE TO TREATMENTS: My exercise routine isn't just a lifestyle choice, it is my core treatment plan. My ability to religiously stick to this plan has been instrumental in managing my progression. Reaching the athletic goals I've set for myself—participating in triathlons, obstacle course races and stair climbs—forces me to adhere to my workout schedule.

FEED OFF THE SUCCESSES OF OTHER PARKINSON'S WARRIORS: I seek out and connect with others who I call fellow "Parkinson's warriors." These are people who approach their own battles with Parkinson's with a similar attitude and are thriving. Witnessing their successes gives me confidence that I can achieve a similar outcome.

KEEP A POSITIVE ATTITUDE: I strive to approach every day with a positive outlook, fighting off any negative feelings of self-pity or self-doubt about my ability to navigate the journey. A positive attitude is a powerful tool—it will help you cope better with your symptoms and respond more effectively to any challenges you face.

DEAL WITH SETBACKS WITH RESILIENCE: I manage my Parkinson's with a problem-solving mindset, viewing any setback not as a failure, but as a challenge to be overcome. If I encounter a potential new symptom, my immediate response is to *understand* it. What is its cause? Is it Parkinson's-related? And most important, how can I deal with it as effectively as possible? This approach yields a deep sense of resilience, enabling me to fight through periods where my current symptoms (typically tremors) might become more noticeable.

REDUCE STRESS AND ANXIETY: Parkinson's can bring on mental and physical strain given the unpredictability of symptoms and other associated factors. I notice an increase in my tremor when I'm anxious, for example. Conversely, when I am preoccupied with something fun and distracting, I can go an extra three to four hours without my next dose of medication. Studies have shown that a positive outlook has neuroprotective effects, whereas chronic stress is damaging to overall health.[7]

MAINTAIN AN OVERALL HEALTHY LIFESTYLE: I strive to optimize my overall wellness. This includes maintaining a healthy diet, embracing low-toxicity living, prioritizing good sleep and more. This dedication ensures that I'm in the best physical and mental shape possible as I battle Parkinson's (more on this in Chapter 5). It gives me a crucial edge in all my endeavors and ensures that I have the energy I need to stay committed to my exercise routine and remain focused on delaying the progression of Parkinson's.

EXPERT INSIGHT
Daniel Corcos on Attitude

Dr. Daniel M. Corcos, PhD, is a professor of Physical Therapy & Human Movement Sciences at Northwestern University's Feinberg School of Medicine. His research focuses on developing exercise interventions to improve quality of life, mobility and cognition and to slow disease progression in people with Parkinson's.

Q: How does attitude impact a person's approach to managing Parkinson's?

DR. CORCOS: The right attitude can make all the difference, but it's not one-size-fits-all. Some individuals are naturally goal-driven and engaged in managing their health, while others may find it harder to take that first step. The encouraging news is that change *is* possible. I try to share the evidence in a way that makes the benefits of exercise undeniable—so even if someone's reluctant, they can see the value and start to make changes. It really comes down to taking ownership and setting priorities. For many, it starts with small steps that build confidence and momentum over time.

Q: Can you talk a little more about the concept of taking ownership?

DR. CORCOS: Sure. Despite the compelling evidence to exercise, some people struggle to take ownership of their exercise regimen. Fortunately, there are other options—for example, getting a personal trainer shares the ownership of managing workouts with the trainer. But that can be expensive. Similarly, a physical therapist can share ownership with you, and it might be covered by insurance. You meet with your therapist once a week and they guide you through a routine.

Q: You also mentioned prioritization. Can you speak more about that?

DR. CORCOS: Once you take ownership, it comes down to prioritization. If exercise is low on your list of priorities, then it's going to slip more often than not. If the single most important thing in your life is managing your health, then that gets plugged into your calendar first and doesn't get deferred. But it requires motivation and good time management.

Q: Are there other sources of motivation to help people take ownership?

DR. CORCOS: Yes. Another source of motivation is family. If you don't take care of yourself, your health will degrade and you will become a burden to your family. The motivation becomes, "If you won't do it for yourself, do it for your loved ones." Another source can be the social accountability of group classes or friend groups in workout apps, where you urge each other on. In a class setting, fellow participants might reach out if they notice you've missed a few sessions, providing additional motivation.

Q: Any parting thoughts on attitude and motivation?

DR. CORCOS: I encourage all people—with or without Parkinson's—to focus on healthspan, which is the period of a person's life during which they are healthy and living well. That's in contrast to *life*span, which is the total number of years a person lives. Healthspan emphasizes not just living longer, but living better. I believe that can be a source of motivation.

BUILDING YOUR SELF-EFFICACY

Everyone possesses some degree of self-efficacy. Our challenge when living with Parkinson's is to build on it and channel it in ways that help us better manage our journey. Bandura developed a scientifically based process for enhancing self-efficacy as part of his research in the 1970s.

STEP ONE is to *set a series of challenging goals*, each enhancing the belief that you can achieve the next. This creates the experience of mastery, which is the foundation of having a strong sense of self-belief. I continually set goals for myself by completing challenging athletic events, such as triathlons and obstacle course races. And I seek out advocacy efforts, which include receiving sponsorship commitments from elected officials on Parkinson's-related legislation. The more I meet these goals, the more my motivation and confidence grow. This goal-oriented approach has been the foundation of building self-efficacy for me.

STEP TWO is to *identify role models to emulate*, such as one or more people living with Parkinson's who are managing their lives well. Seeing others in a similar situation succeed through their determined efforts raises the belief that we, too, can overcome the specific challenges we face. Hearing stories of people who have been living with Parkinson's for more than 20 years and are still living well or hearing stories of 70-year-olds with Parkinson's completing marathons gives me confidence that I can live with a high quality of life well into the future.

STEP THREE is to *seek positive reinforcement and encouragement*, strengthening the belief that we have what it takes to succeed. Socializing with others with Parkinson's who embody the same attitude and approach—and getting support and encouragement from my family and friends—fuels my confidence that I can win my personal battle. I post summaries and photos of athletic events I complete on social media and send periodic email updates to my family and friends. The responses I get back are a big source of motivation to keep up my fight.

🌷 LIVING PARKINSON'S
Sara Whittingham ('Yoda')

ESCAPING THE DARK SIDE WITH GRATITUDE

Sara Whittingham, a physician and U.S. Air Force veteran, is also a mother and endurance athlete based in Aurora, Ohio.

U.S. Air Force Academy graduate Sara Whittingham, known by the call sign "Yoda," considers attitude a pivotal force in managing her Parkinson's journey. Following her diagnosis in 2020, Sara describes succumbing to "the dark side": she experienced significant anxiety, depression, weight gain and poor sleep, leading her to envision a future defined by a "downward trajectory with no control." She recalls telling her classmates from the Air Force Academy "to prepare to help me decorate my wheelchair or my walker at our next reunion in five years."

A crucial turning point emerged during a month-long leave from work. This break enabled her to step back and redefine her path. At the time, Sara serendipitously discovered a handout about a research study investigating the effects of cycling on Parkinson's. To her amazement, the primary researcher was Dr. Jay Alberts, who she had briefly met months before her diagnosis. She enrolled in the study, which provided a Peloton bike and regular encouragement. It ignited a profound shift.

Another motivating factor was the people she met in the study who had been living with Parkinson's for ten years and were still exercising. That got rid of her mental image of requiring a walker in a couple of years. As she increasingly rode the bike, she began to feel better and like "the Force" was being awakened in her.

Beyond exercise, gratitude became a cornerstone of her transformed attitude. She identifies three key influences: observing friends' gratitude posts on Facebook, which uplifted her spirits; learning about "the healing power of gratitude" in a video by her church president; and internalizing Michael J. Fox's philosophy that "with gratitude, optimism is sustainable."

Another deeply personal experience was reconnecting with a pilot she had once grounded 20 years prior due to a medical condition. He was now a general, and his humble gratitude for how his own challenges had made him a better leader resonated with Sara.

As her physical state improved with training, her confidence grew, too. "The more I rode the bike, the better I felt. I was riding it for an hour at a time and thought, 'I can probably ride the bike for three hours.' Then I thought, 'Maybe I could finish a half IRONMAN®.'"

Sara not only qualified for the IRONMAN 70.3® World Championship, she beat her husband by 45 minutes. She then took it a step further: She finished the 2023 IRONMAN World Championship in Kona, Hawaii, proving that nothing can stop you if you have the right attitude.

This carefully cultivated positive attitude propelled Sara into taking on a powerful role as an advocate and motivational speaker. She leveraged her IRONMAN journey and shared it on platforms like *The Today Show* and *Women's Health* magazine to raise awareness about the impact that exercise has on Parkinson's. Her core message: Individuals with Parkinson's don't need to be on a downward trajectory—they *can* take control of this disease by adopting a positive attitude.

THE POWER OF SHORT-TERM GOALS

I have a short attention span, and I thrive when I can achieve a series of short-term goals as part of a larger effort. In contrast, I often get frustrated with long-term activities that don't provide frequent wins. This short-term goal-setting approach has been the key that has driven my efforts and fed my motivation, both in life and in my Parkinson's battle.

When I was in graduate school, I had a difficult time staying motivated when facing a multi-year PhD thesis project. I felt much more comfortable on projects that had milestones in months rather than years. After a while, I changed direction—I focused on my Master's degree, completing it on schedule and graduating to the business world, where there was more focus on shorter-term goals.

Since then, I've become pretty good at setting stretch-yet-achievable goals that I can use as "destinations on a larger journey" or "battles to win in my long-term war with Parkinson's." The satisfaction I get in meeting these goals feeds my confidence and motivates me to move on to the next one.

If Moment One sparked the flame in me,
each goal I reach adds fuel to the fire.

I motivate myself to exercise by setting goals to compete in athletic events that will challenge me every few months. You can do the same. It should be a goal that makes sense for you: You might sign up for a 5K walk or run, complete a yoga or dance class or just push yourself a little further than you have in the past. Your goal can be as simple as accomplishing something new—aim for whatever supports you in your battle with Parkinson's and motivates you.

I'll be sharing more ideas for building self-efficacy throughout *Living Parkinson's* because it's an underlying theme in the strategies that follow. In our journey to beat Parkinson's, self-efficacy provides both the motivation (the fuel) and the goal-oriented approach (the structure).

What You Can Do: Build Momentum with Goals

Start building your *Living Parkinson's* plan now: Set a few short-term attainable goals that you can use as quick doses of motivation, then use those successes to build confidence and take control of your journey.

⚲ EXPERT INSIGHT
Jenna Deidel on the PD SELF® Program

Jenna Deidel is the Director of Programs & Community Impact at the Davis Phinney Foundation, based in Colorado.

Q: Could you start with a little background on the Davis Phinney Foundation and its mission?

JENNA DEIDEL: The Davis Phinney Foundation was founded in 2004 with the mission to help people with Parkinson's live well today. While other organizations focus heavily on research and the search for a cure, the Foundation has always prioritized the day-to-day needs of individuals and families affected by Parkinson's. That mission was borne out of Davis Phinney's own experience. Diagnosed at 40, the former Olympic cyclist was advised to rest, a suggestion he found unacceptable. He and his wife, Connie Carpenter Phinney, channeled that frustration into creating a foundation that empowers people to take a proactive role in their health through education, connection and inspiration.

Q: Could you talk about PD SELF, particularly the emphasis it puts on self-efficacy?

JENNA DEIDEL: We acquired the program and brought it under our banner in 2023. PD SELF focuses on building self-efficacy: the belief that you can set goals, take action and influence your own outcomes. For many, the transition from diagnosis to meaningful action is daunting. PD SELF is designed to help people move through that early stage by building tools and skills like goal-setting, self-awareness and emotional regulation. It addresses not just the person with Parkinson's but also care partners, helping the whole support system feel more empowered. These tools are foundational and can be used throughout life with Parkinson's.

Q: What makes the PD SELF program such a good fit for the Foundation?

JENNA DEIDEL: PD SELF aligns with the Foundation's mission of helping people live well with Parkinson's today. It's grounded in research and has proven results, particularly when it comes to confidence in managing ups and downs, avoiding discouragement, communicating with doctors and fostering emotional well-being. What I find most compelling, however, is that participants have reported positive outcomes even years after completing the program. It's a testament to the way it can impact people over time and improve quality of life for the long haul.

Q: What are the plans for enhancing PD SELF?

JENNA DEIDEL: Our first goal is to get people moving through the program again on a regular basis, which we plan to do primarily through virtual delivery. Long-term, we plan to develop a version of the program for people in the mid and later stages of Parkinson's, when symptoms may change and relationships can become more affected by changing support needs. It's our strong belief that the tools of self-efficacy are relevant at all stages of life with Parkinson's, and we want to equip as many people as we can to build their "self-efficacy force," as program founder Diane Cook likes to say.

DEFINING VICTORY: YOUR OBJECTIVE

I'd like to close out this chapter with what I believe is a crucial step in the *Living Parkinson's* process. Self-efficacy is based on *short-term goals*, yes, but these goals should all roll up into a single vision: your *objective*. I encourage you to begin your efforts by defining your objective—what is your definition of victory and when is your fight over? My objective, which I'll reference throughout *Living Parkinson's*, is:

*Living my best life and keeping Parkinson's at bay
until I'm free from its impact.*

This crystalizes my personal battle. I want to make the most of every day, doing everything I can to slow my Parkinson's progression and support the efforts to find a long-term solution. My battle ends when Parkinson's no longer has any meaningful impact on my daily life, which could take any number of forms. That's when I can declare victory.

What You Can Do: Define Your Objective

Ask yourself: "What does 'winning' look like on my Parkinson's journey?" If it will help you, post what winning looks like wherever you can use it as motivation. Your objective will be the North Star in your journey in that everything you add to your plan should align with your core objective.

Conclusion

Attitude isn't just the starting point—it's the fuel that powers every step of your Parkinson's journey. The moment you take ownership of that journey, everything changes. Whether it centers on building self-efficacy with short-term goals or reframing setbacks as opportunities, your mindset can become one of your best weapons. Choose to live each day with purpose, because your mindset starts with your attitude—and the right frame of mind can jumpstart you on a new path in your battle.

Looking Ahead: Strategy #2 – Knowledge

With the right mindset, you've taken the first step toward fighting back. In the next chapter, we'll talk about why knowledge is power and how the right attitude combined with education can help you take control of your Parkinson's journey.

TAKEAWAYS/ACTION PLANS

CHAPTER 2

KNOWLEDGE
Take Control Through Learning

Every bit of knowledge is another weapon in your fight. Learn like your life depends on it—because it does.

WHAT YOU'LL LEARN IN THIS CHAPTER

▶ Why knowledge is the foundation of an effective Parkinson's strategy

▶ A structured approach to building your personal learning plan

▶ How to identify credible, practical sources of information

▶ Smart tools and tech tips to stay current efficiently

▶ The power of expert insight and how to build your own network of advisors

In *The Art of War*, Sun Tzu wrote, "If you know your enemy … you need not fear." Applying Sun Tzu's wisdom to personal health, the first step in managing your health is understanding what you're facing. That's the focus of this chapter: how you can educate yourself and keep up-to-date with the latest information to put yourself in the best position to win your Parkinson's battle.

By educating myself on what to expect in my Parkinson's journey, I've maintained focus, kept a positive attitude and pushed my limits in athletic events without injury. Knowledge has empowered me to control my progression by identifying and addressing new symptoms—and consequently safeguarding my quality of life.

ANOTHER PROBLEM TO SOLVE

As far back as I can remember, I have been a problem-solver. As a teen, I built electronic devices from schematics as a hobby. In my 20s, I performed maintenance on my car using reference books. And since I've been a homeowner, I perform repairs around the house by reviewing how-to videos and then applying what I've learned.

Living your best life with a neurodegenerative disease like Parkinson's demands a commitment to continuous learning.

I've always enjoyed the challenge of solving problems: clearly defining an objective, gathering and analyzing information, investigating options, selecting a solution and building an action plan. And when dealing with a long-term challenge, the process never ends—it's a cycle that repeats itself. While executing your action plan, if you learn something new (and you usually do), you circle back to reevaluate your options and possibly choose a better solution based on the new information.

The more complex the problem, the more rewarding the outcome. This is still the basis of what I do at work and at home;

the process often leads me to whiteboards or scratch pads packed with notes.

Living your best life with a neurodegenerative disease like Parkinson's demands a commitment to continuous learning. It's ironic that the same organ affected by Parkinson's—the brain—is a key tool in fighting the disease. Education is never-ending! I've found it goes hand in hand with attitude. They are inseparable. Learning more about Parkinson's drives a proactive attitude toward disease management, and a proactive attitude (and self-efficacy) drives the desire to learn more. These two pillars are the foundation for many of the empowering strategies in *Living Parkinson's.*

A Gold Mine of Information

We are lucky to live in a world where we have access to more information than we can possibly consume. It's a bigger challenge to sift through all the information that arrives in our email inboxes than it is to search for an answer to a specific question. Imagine trying to keep up-to-date on the latest Parkinson's information and research 20 or 30 years ago!

If you're old enough to remember a time before the internet, think about it: How *would* you stay up-to-date on the most recent news? Where would you have gone to find that information? How long would it have taken? Today we're in an infinitely better position to access the insights we need to manage our condition.

As you may have done, I've educated myself through books (many bought used online), informative websites, free online courses and a vibrant network of fellow Parkinson's warriors, doctors and researchers. Emails, newsletters, webinars, social media groups and research articles deliver a continuous stream of vital information. I dedicate several hours a week to consume and synthesize Parkinson's-related news and research. This commitment empowers me to manage my journey with greater success than I would have ever thought possible.

MY PARKINSON'S CURRICULUM: THREE KEY LEARNING ZONES

After my diagnosis, I approached my Parkinson's education with a problem-solving mindset. That led me to create an educational structure with three learning zones, each building on the one before it:

1. Understanding the basics of how the brain works.

2. Learning everything about Parkinson's: its symptoms, causes, progression and treatments.

3. Keeping up-to-date on current research and future possibilities.

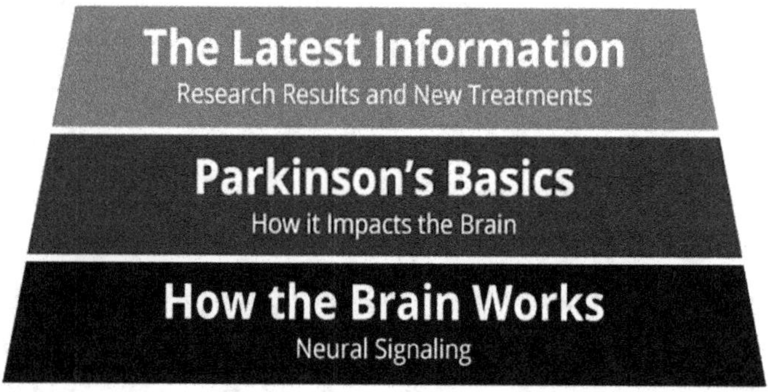

Think of these as three tiers: master the basics, manage the now and monitor the future.

LEARNING ZONE ONE: HOW THE BRAIN WORKS

Before I could understand the impact of Parkinson's, I needed to know how a functioning brain worked. This led me to the field of neuroscience: the study of the brain, spinal cord and nerves. I started by learning all that I could about the topic, which included taking portions of a free online medical neuroscience course from Duke University through Coursera® (an online learning platform). I even bought the course textbook. I focused only on the lectures covering neural signaling since that's the process that controls movement. It got pretty technical, but because of my science background—I have degrees in electrical engineering and a background in chemistry and physics—I was able to grasp the fundamentals.

After listening to the lectures (it took a few tries), I learned that neural signaling is an electrochemical process. The brain communicates using electrical signals transmitted across a series of neurons. An electrical impulse (an action potential) travels down a neuron, and a chemical neurotransmitter (our friend dopamine) carries the signal across the gap between neurons to the next neuron in the chain (see below).

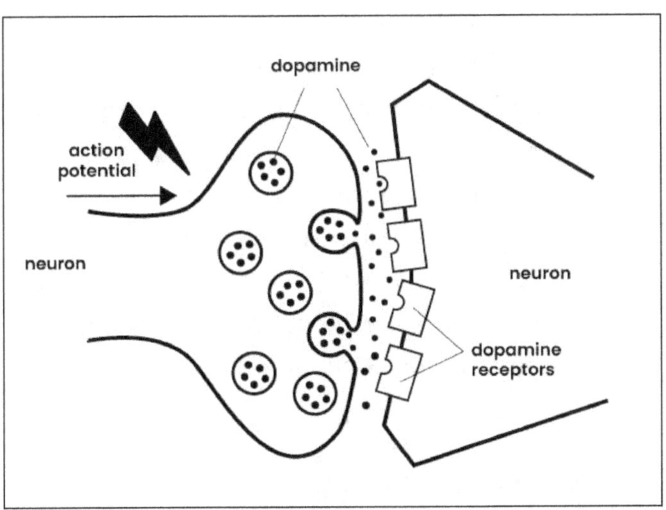

Neural Signaling Process

The transmission continues until the electrical impulse reaches its destination and controls movement. Because Parkinson's reduces available dopamine, the communication process gets disrupted.

Learning these concepts in the medical neuroscience course was challenging—I wouldn't recommend it for everyone. But I also picked up the book *Neuroscience for Dummies* and found that it was an easier read and briefly covered the same topics. If you're curious about how the brain and nervous system work, there's a (very) small section *in Neuroscience for Dummies* that describes it.

Of course, anything you read on neuroscience will contain a lot of content *not* related to neural signaling or Parkinson's, like the senses and memory. But focusing on neural signaling will give you a good basic understanding of the system affected by Parkinson's.

LEARNING ZONE TWO: HOW PARKINSON'S AFFECTS THE BRAIN

Once you have a better handle on how neural signaling works, you can move on to learning more about the details of Parkinson's—starting with how it disrupts the normal signaling process and the possible genetic and environmental causes of Parkinson's, to motor and non-motor symptoms and various treatments and medications. Books and websites are helpful here (see Appendix for some suggested websites), and new resources are constantly emerging. Some resources are more advanced than others, so you'll want to find what clicks best for you.

What You Can Do: Design Your Learning Plan

Focus your learning on the symptoms, medications and treatment options that apply to you. Start with your own diagnosis, then build outward. Targeted knowledge means more informed decisions, less information overload and greater peace of mind.

Knowing What to Expect

The more I've learned about the brain and Parkinson's, the better prepared I've been for new symptoms, how to best manage them and how to make my medication as effective as possible.

I now understand why I sometimes get those annoying toe cramps (dystonia) when I exercise with repetitive motion (on a bike or elliptical) and how to manage around them. I also know that my tremor might get worse after a hard workout and that I shouldn't worry about it. Also, I've learned how to time my medications with my protein intake to make them as effective as possible. In the bigger picture, knowing that I don't have any of the genes currently linked to a higher incidence of Parkinson's means my kids have a lower risk.

The Impact of Environmental Factors

Prevailing theories are that some combination of genetic and environmental factors contribute to the onset of Parkinson's. Given that the incidence of Parkinson's is increasing faster than incidences of other neurological diseases, there's a lot of focus on environmental causes.

It's why I've made some modifications to my lifestyle, such as buying organic fruits and vegetables, using natural personal care products and drinking filtered water. This lifestyle is known as "low-toxicity living" (more on this topic in Chapter 5). I feel so strongly about it that I've encouraged my family to do the same—with varying degrees of success.

Exploring Treatments and Strategies

Armed with a basic understanding of how the brain works and how Parkinson's affects it, I moved on to an important topic: options for better managing my condition. To keep up-to-date, I monitor the latest research and social media posts in Parkinson's groups to see what researchers have proven effective, ineffective or inconclusive and what others have found successful, and I try to learn from positive, negative and inconclusive results alike.

For example, when I read about a dietary modification or supplement with mixed results, I do more research and follow my "No Harm Strategy"—if something might help but won't hurt, I'll consider it.

I've read mixed results pertaining to dietary changes like reducing dairy and taking curcumin as a supplement. Since neither has been shown to have negative effects, I've reduced my dairy intake and started taking a moderate-dose curcumin supplement. Learning the significant impact that exercise could have on slowing progression (more on that in Chapter 4) has changed my life. And I continue to research the latest updates about what exercises work best and then add them to my routine.

While I look at a variety of sources, I weigh them very differently, focusing most of my attention on scientific results from research institutions. Many individuals post on social media about tactics (particularly supplements) that have helped them. While I don't doubt their sincerity, I always look for scientific support before considering any tactic discussed on social media.

What You Can Do: Stick to Science-Backed Sources

If something sounds too good to be true, it probably is. And always consult with your doctor—never experiment alone.

LEARNING ZONE THREE:
STAYING ABREAST OF LATEST TRENDS

Recent research (including studies from the NIH) has taught me about the gut-brain connection in Parkinson's. Newsletters from

The Michael J. Fox Foundation keep me updated on the latest information, like the breakthrough (in 2024) on the diagnostic test for Parkinson's (the alpha-synuclein assay). I also keep informed about new medications such as timed-release options, continuous infusion therapies (think insulin pumps with dopamine) and more effective versions of existing medications.

While I don't need advanced treatments like deep brain stimulation (DBS), I'm always interested in their efficacy, risks and side effects (It never hurts to be prepared, right?). I also monitor treatments on the horizon like ultrasound, infrared light therapy, alpha-synuclein antibodies and stem cells.

Besides increasing my knowledge base about Parkinson's, learning about the progress and positive results shown by these and other potential treatments is uplifting. Planning for the future is helpful, even if some of these options aren't available today. And it's encouraging to know we're closer to new treatments!

EXPERT INSIGHT
Ray Dorsey on Education and Prevention

Dr. Ray Dorsey is the Director of the Center for the Brain & Environment at Atria Health and Research Institute. He is widely recognized for his work in Parkinson's disease, particularly his research emphasizing environmental causes and prevention. He co-authored Ending Parkinson's Disease: A Prescription for Action *and most recently* The Parkinson's Plan.

Q: For someone just diagnosed with Parkinson's, what advice would you give them?

DR. DORSEY: The first thing they need to know is that Parkinson's is a highly treatable disease. It's manageable. People with Parkinson's have walked in space, written books, served in the U.S. Senate and earned PhDs. It needs to be viewed as a new chapter that is manageable. And the more you learn about Parkinson's, the more effective you can be in managing it.

Q: Why is it important to educate yourself on Parkinson's?

DR. DORSEY: There is no cure for Parkinson's. But everyone should know how best to manage his or her disease. And they can do that by knowing what causes it. If we know the causes, we can modify our behavior and perhaps slow its progression.

Empowered patients do better. The more people know the reasons why they have a disease, the more informed decisions they can make in managing their condition. They'll have more self-efficacy, independence and control. For example, they can make informed decisions to avoid harmful substances or pollutants that could accelerate its progression.

Q: Can you provide another example of the benefits of education?

DR. DORSEY: Sure. It can help decrease the likelihood that their children develop the disease. One role of parents, if they have a disease like Parkinson's, is to do everything they can to help prevent their children getting it. There is a 2X increased risk for first-degree relatives to get Parkinson's. This could be from genetic causes or because people vary in their breakdown of toxic chemicals, just like people vary in their breakdown of medicines. And some people might be slower to break down certain toxins or have an underlying genetic susceptibility that maybe not all of us have. Understanding this susceptibility could enable parents to shield their children from it and reduce their risk.

Q: Speaking of education, what can people learn from reading your book, *The Parkinson's Plan?*

DR. DORSEY: Everyone wants to prevent or possibly slow the disease's progression. Our book offers 25 specific recommendations to do that. These are changes that are readily accessible to the vast majority of people in their everyday lives. Taking specific measures like washing fruits and vegetables is a great example.

BENEFITS OF BEING INFORMED

Knowledge is power, especially when you're navigating Parkinson's. For me, making education a priority has been a cornerstone of how I manage my condition. Here are some ways that education has helped me and can make a real difference for you.

EMPOWERING YOU TO TAKE CONTROL AND PROACTIVELY MANAGE YOUR CONDITION: A deeper understanding of Parkinson's enables you to take greater ownership of your condition. You'll better equip yourself to make well-informed decisions about your treatment strategies, including medications, lifestyle adjustments and more. It sharpens your ability to identify new symptoms or subtle shifts in your overall disease progression.

I've adapted my regimen in meaningful ways, guided by what I've learned and continue to discover about Parkinson's. For example, I've incorporated specific exercises like the speed bag and heavy bag into my workouts, made thoughtful dietary choices like eliminating dairy and strategically adjusted the timing of my medications.

HELPING YOU COMMUNICATE WITH YOUR HEALTHCARE TEAM: The time you get with your doctor is a precious resource, and maximizing its value is essential. I see my appointments as a

50/50 split between consulting with an expert and undergoing a physical examination. I dedicate the initial portion of each appointment with my movement disorder specialist to discuss current research and any changes I have observed in my condition. The more educated and prepared you are when meeting with your healthcare team, the better questions you can ask, which leads to more meaningful discussions and more value from your time together. This empowers you to become a more effective advocate for yourself.

IMPROVING TREATMENT ADHERENCE: Understanding how certain medications, therapies or lifestyle changes affect your symptoms and why doctors recommend them improves treatment adherence. It also enables you to recognize their effectiveness or early warning signs if they're not producing the desired results. My knowledge of the medications I take helps me optimize the timing of them and identify unwanted side effects at the earliest possible stage (such as the impulsive behaviors I experienced with dopamine agonists).

EXPANDING YOUR NETWORK: Collecting more information about Parkinson's often leads to finding support groups, online communities and patient advocacy organizations. Engaging with others who share similar experiences not only provides access to a wealth of practical information but also can be a powerful source of motivation and mutual empowerment.

KEEPING YOU UPDATED ON NEW TREATMENTS: The landscape of disease and medical research is constantly evolving. Staying informed enables you to remain current on new treatments, clinical trials and significant advancements that hold the potential to improve your long-term outcome. Following the latest research has educated me on potential therapies such as alpha-synuclein antibodies, ultrasound therapies, wearables, stem cells and more—building a sense of hope and optimism toward future possibilities.

REDUCING THE ANXIETY THAT COMES WITH UNCERTAINTY: Dealing with the unknown associated with a neurodegenerative disease can be very unsettling. Studies—including those summarized by The Michael J. Fox Foundation—show that stress worsens Parkinson's symptoms such as tremors, rigidity and anxiety.

Learning about Parkinson's can serve as a powerful antidote to this anxiety by preparing you for the future and removing unnecessary stress. It also equips you with the knowledge you need to navigate the vast amount of information available and to discern credible sources from any misinformation or negative perspectives you might encounter.

What You Can Do: Prepare for Doctor Visits

Bring a written list of questions to your next doctor's visit along with a notepad to take notes. It's easy to forget what's said—writing things down helps you remember key details and ensures all your questions get answered.

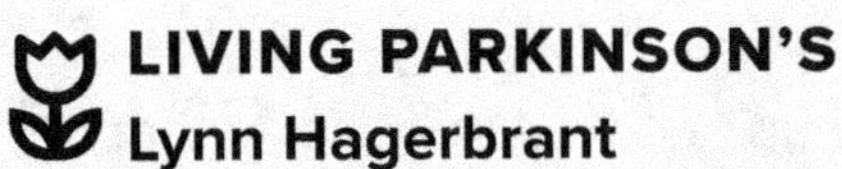 **LIVING PARKINSON'S**
Lynn Hagerbrant

KNOWLEDGE IS HOPE AND A SEAT AT THE TABLE

Lynn Hagerbrant, a retired cardiac intensive care nurse and co-founder and chairman of the board of Parkinson's Body & Mind, is based in Greenwich, CT.

Lynn Hagerbrant is a retired nurse with a background in critical care. But her medical training didn't fully prepare her for Parkinson's—she rarely encountered it, and she associated it with elderly patients. Her early mental image of Parkinson's was the stereotypical one: an old man hunched over a cane. When she was diagnosed with Parkinson's herself, she struggled to accept it. "I respectfully disagree with the diagnosis," she told her neurologist. "There's no way I could have Parkinson's."

At first, Lynn rejected the idea of learning more about the disease. "I didn't want to be educated," she admits. "That was part of my denial." But as her journey progressed, so did her mindset. Over time, she began to embrace the power of knowledge—not just for herself, but for the larger community. She came to see education as a tool of empowerment rather than a burden.

Lynn began to approach Parkinson's with courage and a desire to improve outcomes. Learning about the disease—its symptoms, progression, treatments and nuances—gave her not only clarity, but a renewed sense of control. And, in her words, "learning about Parkinson's provides hope by understanding the progress being made in research and the opportunity to live the best life possible."

Perhaps most importantly, gaining more knowledge changed her relationship with her medical team. "When you don't understand your condition, it's easy to feel powerless," she says. "You show up and wait to be told what to do." However, as Lynn grew more informed, she saw herself as an active partner, not a passive patient. She asked better questions. She understood her medications. She made more thoughtful decisions about her care.

Education gave her a seat at the table—and a voice, too.

Lynn also sees the power of local support groups, where learning isn't a one-way street: Sharing knowledge and experiences with others creates a powerful feedback loop. Seeing others navigate the same challenges helps her feel more equipped and turns group meetings into a source of strength, perspective and practical wisdom.

Lynn didn't stop at her own learning. She co-founded Parkinson's Body & Mind (PBM), a nonprofit organization that brings accessible, evidence-based programs to people with Parkinson's. PBM brings researchers and patients together, fostering education in the broader community. The program integrates exercise, education and community support to help others take ownership of their own Parkinson's journeys.

Today, Lynn is a passionate advocate for Parkinson's awareness, education and patient empowerment. Her unique blend of clinical knowledge and lived experience enables her to bridge the gap between the medical community and those living with the disease. She believes deeply that patients who understand their condition can help shape their care, not just receive it. "When you take the time to learn," she says, "you shift the power. You're no longer just surviving—you're leading."

TRUSTED SOURCES THAT DELIVER

As I've managed my journey with Parkinson's, I appreciate the importance of having reliable sources of information. It helps me navigate the complexities and make informed choices. There are incredible resources out there, and tapping into them can empower you, too. Here are some I rely on to keep me educated:

Major Parkinson's Organizations and News Websites

The major Parkinson's organizations offer a wealth of information on every aspect of the disease alongside complementary resources like webinars, educational conferences and opportunities to connect with others through meet-ups, both local and virtual.

Subscribing to their email updates is a simple yet powerful way to ensure you stay informed about the latest developments. Explore these organizations based on your location (See Appendix or go to livingparkinsons.com for a list).

One source, the PD Avengers Parkinson's News page (www.pdavengers.com/parkinsons-news), has become part of my daily routine. I review it almost every morning to see the latest Parkinson's news from around the world. I've found it to be among the best ways to stay on top of what's happening. I encourage you to bookmark this page and keep it accessible in your own browser.

Niche/Focused Resources and Communities

As I've connected with more individuals with Parkinson's, I've learned about additional online resources, most of which are managed by individuals within the community. Many such niche resources exist, and I recommend finding ones that align with your needs: your approach, interests, goals or location. An example that I've found to be valuable is The Parkinson's Fight Club Facebook group. The group approaches Parkinson's with the proactive, positive attitude covered in Chapter 1.

There are many informative Facebook groups dedicated to different aspects of Parkinson's. Some have a more negative tone and focus on life's difficulties; others may promote unverified theories or treatments. I advise you to approach them with caution. Instagram also offers a range of informative and inspiring accounts from both organizations and individuals, but with the same caveat.

Books and More for Deeper Learning

A wide selection of books is available covering topics such as Parkinson's pathophysiology (disease processes), symptoms, treatments, medication, exercise as a therapeutic approach and more. A quick search on Amazon can provide you with some of the bestsellers and highest-rated books on a specific topic.

You also can search for articles on more detailed topics (e.g., neuroplasticity) that interest you. For a more complete understanding, consider taking online courses from platforms such as Coursera and edX®. Coursera, for example, is the platform where I audited the Duke University medical neuroscience course.

What You Can Do: Get Started Online

Pick a short list of reliable sources and sign up for their newsletters today. Bookmark them and scan for updates weekly—it's the simplest way to stay informed without being overwhelmed by information overload.

ADVANCED OPTIONS FOR TECHIES

For individuals who are more tech-savvy, here are a few advanced techniques (a.k.a. hacks) for staying informed.

SETTING UP GOOGLE SEARCH ALERTS: I use a Google Alert™ for "Parkinson's" to deliver search results to me weekly on new Parkinson's information. Google Alerts offer a great deal of flexibility, from specific search terms to frequency of delivery. If you're interested in a more specific topic like "Parkinson's ultrasonic therapy," you could set an alert to provide results on that specific search term at whatever frequency is best for you.

USING ARTIFICIAL INTELLIGENCE (AI) AS YOUR RESEARCH ASSISTANT: Artificial intelligence is an exploding field. I have no doubt that by the time this book is published, these examples may be outdated. But today, I rely on Google Gemini™ as my research assistant. For example, I might say, "Summarize the latest research on constipation and Parkinson's disease."

The speed and capacity of these tools to synthesize information is amazing and can be an enormous time-saver. If the initial response is too technical, a follow-up request for clarification in simpler terms such as "Please summarize those results in less technical terms" can yield a more basic explanation. You can enable voice in these tools and literally have a conversation with your AI assistant. I have had many five-minute conversations with Gemini delving into topics I'm looking to learn more about. But be careful and always review the results—AI is an evolving technology, and responses may include mistakes.

CREATING WEBINAR SUMMARIES: I get invited to multiple informative Parkinson's webinars every week. These are a great source of the latest information or updates on specific topics. But attending these live events is time-consuming, and it's hard to tell which ones will benefit me. If I'm not sure about the value of a webinar or I have a scheduling conflict, I'll skip the live event. I can do this because organizers typically record webinars on platforms like YouTube® and send registrants a link to the recording after the event.

You can often download transcripts of these recordings, but if they're unavailable, online services can generate them if provided with the link to the recording. Just google "YouTube transcript extractor" to find these services, enter the link to the recording and then download the transcript. Once you have the transcript, you can upload it to an AI tool and request a summary. I can get a two-page summary of a one-hour webinar in less than a minute. This is a great time-saver for me, and if you're technically savvy, it can be for you, too.

What You Can Do: Create Your First Google Alert

Go to www.google.com/alerts and pick a topic you're interested in, or you can just use "Parkinson's disease." I recommend setting the frequency to "at most once a week" to avoid getting overwhelmed.

BUILDING A NETWORK

One of the best ways to educate yourself about Parkinson's is by connecting with doctors, researchers and others living with it. When I meet with any doctor or member of my care team, I always arrive, pen and paper in hand, with a list of topics I want to discuss and questions I want to ask.

I also take advantage of online patient portals like MyChart® for asking questions between appointments, whether about a supplement I'm considering or a change in symptoms I'm experiencing. I don't hesitate to reach out to researchers I've read about or have seen speaking at a conference or webinar if I have unanswered or follow-up questions.

What You Can Do: Ask Questions

If you have a question for a researcher or speaker, you can usually find their email address with a simple Google search, especially if they're working at an educational institution.

During a recent American Parkinson Disease Association (APDA) conference, the keynote speaker presented his vision for future treatments. At the end of his presentation, he included a slide on actionable steps to take now to address Parkinson's progression. One recommendation was to take creatine for mitochondrial health. Following the presentation, I spoke to him about this recommendation, and based on our discussion, I began incorporating it into my regimen.

Connecting to others with Parkinson's also provides a valuable learning opportunity. I'll often ask others about treatments—exercises, medicines or supplements—they have found helpful. This is particularly valuable as it can provide options that others living with Parkinson's have received from their medical teams. You can view these as "indirect professional second opinions" to take back to your own doctor for discussion.

I've learned about new medications through these connections that I've then explored with my movement disorder specialist, for example. Cultivating what I call your "Parkinson's network" is a recurring theme in this book because of the wealth of knowledge and support it provides.

Conclusion

Knowledge is one of the most powerful tools you have in the fight against Parkinson's. The more you learn, the more empowered, confident and in control you can be. Staying informed can help you make smarter decisions, collaborate more effectively with your care team and better manage your journey.

Looking Ahead: Strategy #3 – Support

Armed with knowledge, you're better prepared to act. But you don't have to go it alone! In the next chapter, we'll talk about building a team to support you in your fight.

TAKEAWAYS/ACTION PLAN

CHAPTER 3

SUPPORT
Build and Strengthen Your Team

No one has to fight Parkinson's alone.
The strength of your support is the
strength of your fight.

WHAT YOU'LL LEARN IN THIS CHAPTER

▶ How to build a comprehensive support team
tailored to your needs

▶ Why your care team should go beyond
just one doctor

▶ How to strengthen your Circle of Support with
family and friends

▶ The power of connecting with the broader
Parkinson's community

▶ The physical and emotional benefits of having
the right support

Everyone's Parkinson's journey is unique; we've established that. But that doesn't mean you'll be going on this journey alone. Now that you've built the right attitude and armed yourself with knowledge, you're ready to choose who to take with you.

YOUR SUPPORT TEAM

It's not an exaggeration to view our life with Parkinson's as a personal war. And in this war, you are the commander-in-chief. You're in charge. And the campaign's success hinges on your decisions. But no one can fight a war without motivated troops and deep intelligence about the enemy.

You'll also need to choose a set of trusted advisers who are experts in their fields. They are your care team of doctors and specialists who provide you with evidence-based medical advice to help you manage your Parkinson's. And to power your campaign, you'll need supplies (fuel, food, equipment) to drive your war machine. That lifeline of support comes from the family and friends you choose to inform about your diagnosis and who go on the journey with you.

Your fellow Parkinson's warriors are the people who are with you in the foxhole, fighting alongside you. They're uniquely qualified to understand the challenges you face, sharing strategies from their own experiences and providing unwavering solidarity.

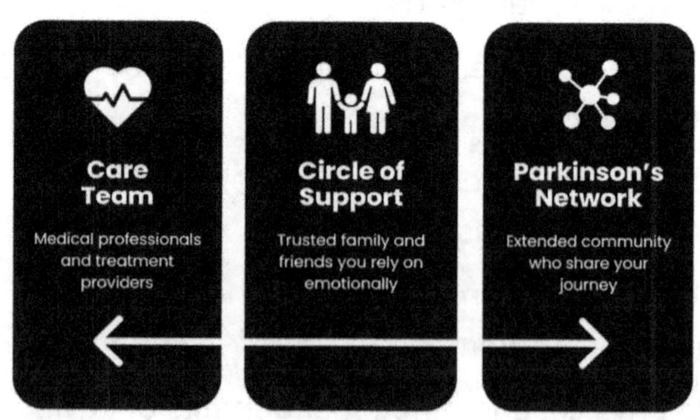

The three groups that form your support team

GROUP ONE: BUILD YOUR CARE TEAM

When my diagnosis was confirmed at Mount Sinai in New York, the doctor recommended I see a local movement disorder specialist at Yale as my primary doctor. That was the first step in building my care team. A Google search led me to a movement disorder specialist who I met for a consultation based on his background, experience and specialty.

I saw that first appointment as a two-way interview—I was evaluating him just as much as he was evaluating me. He needed to *earn* a spot on my care team. I viewed my evaluation of him as, "Do I want to make this doctor my most trusted advisor on one of the most important journeys of my life?" I liked his approach and decided he would be the key advisor on my care team. We currently meet every four months.

What You Can Do: Find the Right Doctor

Search for a movement disorder specialist (MDS) in your area or for a neurologist if an MDS isn't available. A movement disorder specialist is a neurologist with advanced training in conditions like Parkinson's. Prepare questions to evaluate whether he or she is the right doctor for you. Focus on expertise, communication style and how well they understand your goals.

ADD MULTIPLE PERSPECTIVES

In 2023, at a local Parkinson's conference, I saw a presentation by a movement disorder specialist who was advocating for a holistic treatment approach, focusing on the "whole" patient instead of just the Parkinson's. An integrated approach to care—

that intrigued me. I was interested to see how she'd approach my condition.

I reached out to my primary, who had no problem giving me a referral. I made it clear that my intention wasn't to question his care but to get another perspective on my diagnosis and treatment. A good physician shouldn't have a problem with this kind of request. If they do, they might not be a team player and right for your care team.

Remember, this is *your* life, *your* battle and *your* team, and you need to do what *you* feel is necessary. I've found that many others in the Parkinson's community also have benefited from consulting multiple movement disorder specialists.

For me, consulting with this specialist was about strategically diversifying my care team and integrating complementary approaches for managing Parkinson's with my current treatment. It also added a new perspective to my team of advisors, all of whom might bring different ideas to the table.

My initial evaluation with the new specialist included a detailed exam plus a comprehensive panel of blood tests—38 in all. I was drawn to anything that offered more insight into my overall health. All of my test results were within normal parameters, apart from a couple of minor readings that were slightly out of range.

Given that this new group practiced an integrated approach to care, I took the opportunity to see their nutritionist. My goal was to optimize my overall wellness. The nutritionist recommended adding one new supplement and removing another, which brought the minor deficiencies in my bloodwork back into the normal range. This has given me peace of mind that I'm in the best possible position to wage my war with Parkinson's.

I also added a physical therapist to my care team. My exercise routine occasionally brings on minor aches and pains, and when they become more persistent, I work with a physical therapist to address them.

Those professionals make up my care team: a primary movement disorder specialist, a second movement disorder specialist and nutritionist in an integrated care group, my primary care doctor and the physical therapist. Being a patient of an integrated care team gives me access to more Parkinson's specialists who can be added to the team if my situation changes.

What You Can Do: Build Your Care Team

Your care team is *your* choice. Don't let any discomfort of asking your primary for a referral or for a second opinion stop you.

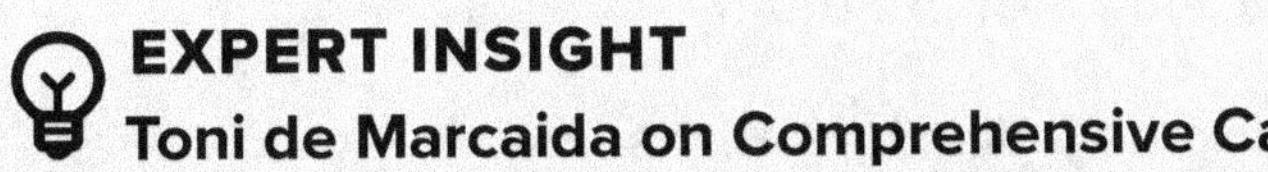

EXPERT INSIGHT
Toni de Marcaida on Comprehensive Care

Dr. J. Antonelle "Toni" de Marcaida, MD, is a movement disorder specialist at Hartford HealthCare and a leader in developing one of the most comprehensive Parkinson's care programs in the region.

Q: What is comprehensive care in medicine?

DR. DE MARCAIDA: Comprehensive care refers to a holistic and thorough approach to care that brings together multiple disciplines—neurology, physical therapy, occupational therapy, speech therapy, mental health, social work, other medical subspecialists and even wellness programs—under one umbrella to care for the whole person. It's not just about treating the motor symptoms of Parkinson's, but also enhancing one's overall sense of well-being while addressing other aspects affected by the disease.

Q: Within a comprehensive care approach, how does integrative medicine (employing non-Western therapies) fit in?

DR. DE MARCAIDA: Integrative medicine isn't about replacing your neurologist, it's about expanding your toolbox. For some people with Parkinson's, options like acupuncture, massage therapy or naturopathic treatments can help manage symptoms that medications don't fully address, like fatigue, pain or digestive issues. When done thoughtfully, they can enhance quality of life. Today, more than 60% of people with Parkinson's tend to seek out complementary therapies. When that's the case, we feel it's always best done with the guidance of a physician rather than independently.

Q: What are some indications that someone would benefit from a comprehensive care approach?

DR. DE MARCAIDA: I believe that everyone would benefit from this approach. It becomes even more crucial when struggling with more of the nonmotor symptoms of Parkinson's, such as cognition, mood, sleep, gastrointestinal or bladder issues—or challenges with balance, speech, swallowing or daily activities. At that point, there may be a greater need for a broader support team to manage these more effectively.

Q: Any examples of how this approach made a difference in someone's care?

DR. DE MARCAIDA: Absolutely. I have so many people who express to us how the comprehensive care we provide has changed their lives. I've seen it help them overcome depression and anxiety and improve their overall quality of life. Even in more advanced stages of Parkinson's, with coordinated care, they regain confidence, start exercising, and feel hopeful and empowered. A comprehensive care approach can transform people's lives.

Q: What can someone do if they don't have a comprehensive care practice near them?

DR. DE MARCAIDA: Build your own team. You can still see a neurologist, a physical therapist and a speech therapist even if they're not all at one location. Start by educating yourself so you can recognize which symptoms or experiences might actually be part of the disease. Then find a specialist who covers that area and bring them onto your team. Ask your providers to collaborate. Bring your own records. The building may not be labeled a "Comprehensive Care Center," but you can still advocate for yourself to receive integrated care.

Who Can Be on Your Integrated Team

A movement disorder specialist or neurologist should be at the core of your team, but other professionals can play vital roles, too. While there are many options, your team will likely only contain those professionals whose areas of expertise match your needs. Here's a snapshot of the most common specialists and how they might support you:

SPECIALIST	ROLE IN PARKINSON'S CARE
Movement Disorder Specialist	Diagnosis, medication, long-term treatments
Primary Care Doctor	General health monitoring, referrals to specialists
Physical Therapist	Mobility, balance, strength training
Occupational Therapist	Daily living adaptations, home modifications
Speech-Language Pathologist	Speech and swallowing issues
Neuropsychologist	Manages cognitive, memory, behavioral issues
Social Worker/Psychologist	Emotional and mental health support
Exercise Professional	Leads programs like boxing, dance and cycling
Nutritionist/Dietitian	Diet optimization, gut health
Neurosurgeon	Deep Brain Stimulation (DBS) surgery
Urologist	Urinary symptoms common in Parkinson's
Gastroenterologist	Constipation or delayed stomach emptying
Pharmacist	Manages medications, timings and interactions

If you add any specialists to your care team, try to find ones with a focus on Parkinson's, given the specific symptoms that can occur (e.g., complex digestive issues). You can also include complementary therapies—such as acupuncture, mindful movement and massage therapy—that some practices incorporate alongside conventional care.

The specific composition of your team should always reflect your individual needs. Your team should include any professionals who you believe will help you manage your Parkinson's symptoms. There are no limits and there is no right or wrong. This is *your* team! Seek the expertise of any professional who you believe can help you achieve the best possible quality of life.

GROUP TWO: BRING IN FAMILY AND FRIENDS

While your care team provides professional expertise to manage Parkinson's, your emotional support is sustained by those closest to you. Your family and friends may not hold medical degrees, but their presence, belief in you and daily encouragement often play an even more powerful role in your ability to stay motivated and hopeful. According to research from Johns Hopkins Medicine, emotional support from close relationships is strongly linked to better health outcomes in chronic illnesses, including Parkinson's.

Telling My Family

After my diagnosis, my thoughts immediately went to my wife, my four children (who ranged from 19 to 25 years old at the time) and my parents. But determining the right way to tell them without causing undue concern was important to me. And I wanted to be sure I could personally deliver the news and that none of them would hear it from anyone else.

I found a time when we were all together. We sat in a circle in my parents' living room. It was awkward. After all, how often do you call your family together for a "serious meeting"?

Once everyone had quieted down, I came right out and said, "I have something important to talk about. I went to a neurologist for a tremor in my left hand, and he diagnosed me with Parkinson's disease."

This time it was me who spoke those familiar words I had heard from all of my doctors: "Parkinson's does not significantly reduce your lifespan." I did my best to focus on the "positive" aspects, as I didn't want the news to worry my family unnecessarily.

I tried to imagine how I would have felt as a 25-year-old

to hear that my father had Parkinson's. Or even worse, as an 85-year-old to hear that my son had Parkinson's. They all had different reactions; some just had a blank look on their faces. Clearly, no one had been expecting anything like this. Just like someone who's on their own Parkinson's journey, we all process the news of hearing that a loved one has been diagnosed with Parkinson's in our own way.

At our family meeting, some members were more affected than others, but I urged them all not to be overly concerned. I realize now that the image most people have of a person with Parkinson's is someone in an advanced stage who has very pronounced symptoms.

As you may have experienced yourself, telling your family you have a neurodegenerative disease kind of kills the mood for the rest of the day. It felt a little like a dark cloud was following us around for a while. After each family member had gone through their own acceptance period, though, they began to open up about their thoughts and emotions.

USING THEIR WORDS AS MOTIVATION

When I was first diagnosed, my wife immediately began thinking about the future: what life would look like and how to plan for it, assuming she would outlive me or have to take care of me later in life. My kids were shocked. Because I had always lived such a healthy lifestyle, Parkinson's was the last thing they'd expected. They didn't know how to react at first. None of us did.

Zack captured my kids' shared disbelief:

> *"Growing up, you were my biggest role model—someone who could solve any problem or accomplish anything. When I found out you had Parkinson's, my initial reaction was disbelief."*

Melissa's first thoughts turned to legacy:

"I didn't want my children to know you only through stories if you weren't around."

But over time, as they watched how I responded to the diagnosis, each of them found their own version of acceptance—and admiration.

Matt reflected on my renewed sense of purpose:

"Instead of letting it get you down, you turned it into a positive, finding a new purpose and letting it fuel you."

Jake focused on resilience:

"You haven't let it stop you from doing the things that give your life meaning."

Melissa noticed the intensity of my fight:

"Your dedication to fighting Parkinson's is unlike anything I've ever seen. You never rest."

And Zack echoed the core of who they've always known me to be:

"You've never backed down from a challenge. Once you set your mind to beating Parkinson's, I knew there would be no stopping you."

As you can see, we're a close family. Their words and support have become part of the fuel that keeps me moving forward—reminding me every day that I have something worth fighting for and to never give up. And I try to be a role model for them just in case they ever have to face a similar challenge in their lives.

Using Support as Fuel

My family has backed up those words with support. They participate in athletic events with me as *Team Yellen* (although sometimes only after a lot of coaxing from me). Believe it or not, not everyone enjoys spending two-plus hours ankle deep in mud on a Sunday afternoon in an obstacle course race! But they're always encouraging me and cheering me on when they come to watch.

While the energy I get from my kids is like a bolt of lightning when we finish a race together, I don't want to overlook the 24/7 support I get from my wife, Hillary. She's the constant—always there in the background (and often the foreground) encouraging me and reminding me about what really matters. Her steady presence fuels the fight just as much as the big moments do.

My wife and kids have also joined me at Parkinson's events in the community and helped me with fundraising. We've participated as a team in Parkinson's Revolutions—a group spinning class—with teams in both New York and Boston over the past three years. They've even joined me in advocating for the National Act to End Parkinson's with U.S. Senators in their districts (more on advocacy in Chapter 6). It's become something we do together—a family effort that brings us closer.

Beyond my family, I also told my close friends about my Parkinson's, mostly in one-on-one conversations (My script with them was similar to the one I had used for my family). Everyone I've told has supported me in my efforts, but one case particularly stands out. I was at a wedding reception with a college buddy who I don't see very often, and I'll never forget his response when I told him the news.

He put his arm around me and—with the benefit of a few drinks in him—he said:

"If anyone can beat this, you can."

Those words have stuck with me to this day. I have them etched in my brain like a motivational sticker.

Another close friend, after seeing the effort I'd been putting into fighting Parkinson's, said:

"If one of us had to get it, I'm glad it was you. I could never put the effort into the fight that you are."

I took that as a compliment, which was how he intended it. I think about that a lot, too, and I also use his words as motivation.

CREATE YOUR CIRCLE OF SUPPORT

I've been very deliberate about who I bring into my "Circle of Support," because this is the group I rely on for encouragement, emotional support and trust. Trust in particular needs to be part of the criteria for who to include because we all might have some confidentiality associated with our diagnosis. My circle has naturally grown over time as I've chosen to invite more family and friends to join me on my journey. As I look back, I have no regrets about telling anybody.

What You Can Do: Expand Your Circle of Support

Bring people into your Circle of Support who will be the best at fueling your efforts. Focus on those who energize you and support your goals—this is *your* team, and *you* decide who's on it.

Keep the Support Flowing

One reason I refer to this group as my *Circle of Support* is because I continuously communicate with them. Since many of them express an interest in *Team Yellen* activities, I send out periodic emails updating this group on our accomplishments. Each encouraging response I get provides me with a shot of energy to do more. It feels great! I get frequent feedback from family and close friends.

But most gratifying is when I hear from people I wouldn't normally expect to hear from: graduate assistants I've worked with in research studies, professional colleagues I haven't seen in years and distant relatives. It's also incredibly gratifying when people pick up on the nuances of my efforts.

One cousin recently acknowledged my accomplishments and added:

> *"What's really awesome is the lifelong memories you are creating by doing these events with your kids."*

He gets it.

And it's more than just the athletic events—family and friends who live across the country have joined me in advocacy calls with their U.S. Senators to promote the National Plan to End Parkinson's.

The concept of this book came from a writer friend who, after reading my *Team Yellen* update emails, suggested I take on this project. It took multiple tries for him to convince me, as I had never before considered writing a book. The reinforcement I've received from those I've shared early versions of the *Living Parkinson's* with has been so uplifting! I attribute much of what I've done in my Parkinson's efforts to the constant doses of encouragement I get from this group.

The support I've received—even from unexpected places—has helped keep me focused and energized. But there's an ironic flip side, too. Because I've been fortunate to manage my Parkinson's so well to date, I feel like some family and friends occasionally forget I have it. They don't always see the constant work and unrelenting effort it takes to maintain my level of functioning. I remind myself that it's not their fault—it's a byproduct of doing well. But it's also a quiet challenge many of us face: managing the invisible efforts while staying positive. That's why keeping support flowing through regular connection and sharing matters so much.

GROUP THREE:
CONNECT WITH FELLOW WARRIORS

Along with support from family and friends, connecting with others who have Parkinson's offers empathy, motivation and lived experience that no one else can provide. And the Parkinson's community is amazing! I've found the level of camaraderie to be astonishing. It shows the bond that can be built among those with a common fight: Parkinson's warriors who share a similar mindset and approach and truly understand the day-to-day battle.

I have made a concerted effort to meet others in the Parkinson's community—not just others with the disease, but researchers and other experts. Virtually everyone has been receptive, and my interactions have been gratifying. I've built relationships that have grown into friendships.

I look for groups of fellow Parkinson's warriors, people who are facing the disease head-on with the same attitude as me. I've met some inspiring people, both in person and online, including many who are featured in this book. They've done amazing things, from completing IRONMAN races and marathons to raising tens of thousands of dollars—and their stories have deeply inspired me.

What You Can Do: Join a Group

Search for a local or online Parkinson's group
that matches your approach and mindset.
Prioritize positive, active communities—they'll lift
you up and help you stay motivated.

FIND YOUR FIT

There are lots of online and local in-person Parkinson's groups out there. Some are more traditional support groups with a counselor; some are social groups; some are exercise-focused (e.g., dance groups, boxing). Exercise groups are doubly beneficial, providing both camaraderie and encouragement to stick to your exercise routine. There are many excellent websites where you can find these groups—the Appendix includes a list of some of the major organizations.

If you find a group that's the right fit, you can gain incredible encouragement and build lasting relationships, helping you to extend your Circle of Support. These groups often become gateways to even more connections as members introduce you to others and help you expand your Parkinson's network. I've been able to connect with leading researchers and have meaningful conversations with legal and insurance professionals about managing my future, and I've even received invitations to special events hosted by major organizations.

One last comment on support groups: They can also fill the void if—for whatever reason—you don't have the support you need from family and friends. If you're in a situation where you aren't getting the support you need, I encourage you to search out a local group to fill your Circle of Support. Don't fight this battle alone!

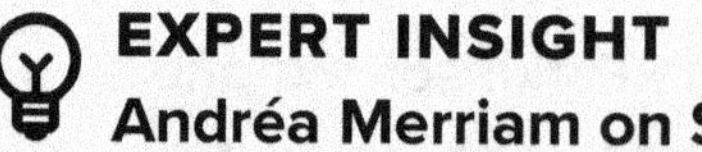

EXPERT INSIGHT
Andréa Merriam on Support Groups

Andréa Merriam is the CEO of PMD Alliance.

Q: What support groups are available for people with Parkinson's?

ANDRÉA MERRIAM: Support groups today take many forms. There are virtual groups as well as traditional in-person gatherings at hospitals, movement disorder clinics and community centers. Some groups are peer-led, while others are facilitated by professionals such as social workers, nurses or counselors. They also vary in structure—some are speaker-based, featuring guest experts, while others are discussion-focused, where members share experiences and support one another. More recently, activity-based and social formats have emerged, from walk-and-talk sessions to outdoor adventures like rafting or cycling.

Q: What are some of the benefits people get from support groups?

ANDRÉA MERRIAM: Support groups offer space to express fears and frustrations—a reminder that "when it can be mentioned, it can be managed." They provide firsthand advice on everything from physical therapists to neurologists. The most profound benefit, though, is community. Having people who "get it" reduces isolation and builds belonging, which is essential when navigating Parkinson's.

Q: What makes a Parkinson's support group truly effective?

ANDRÉA MERRIAM: The key ingredient is psychological safety—a place where participants can be authentic and honest without judgment. PMD Alliance trains volunteer leaders and provides resources to help them create these safe, inclusive spaces. A group works best when members feel comfortable showing up as they are—on or off, hopeful or struggling—and know they'll be met with understanding.

Q: What advice would you give to someone who's hesitant about joining a group?

ANDRÉA MERRIAM: Try one—or several. Each group has its own personality and culture. Reach out to leaders beforehand or attend a virtual session to observe quietly. Not all groups are alike, and the right fit makes all the difference.

Q: How have virtual or hybrid support formats changed accessibility or participation?

ANDRÉA MERRIAM: Online groups have made participation easier and more inclusive. They enable people to find others with similar backgrounds because they offer a wider reach, something that might be hard to find when limited to a specific location.

Q: How does the work of PMD Alliance champion a sense of community?

ANDRÉA MERRIAM: PMD Alliance's mission is to connect people to the Parkinson's community and create resources that enhance care. Support groups are central to our mission. We offer training, online and in-person classes, videos and manuals, along with mentorship to inspire and equip group leaders. The goal is simple but powerful: help every person feel seen, heard and empowered through connection.

Grow Your Network

Your Parkinson's network can grow in many ways. One meaningful example for me began with a research study I joined in 2023 at Teachers College at Columbia University. I made the effort to connect with the program director, and a few months later, she referred me to a team that was creating an exercise brochure for The Michael J. Fox Foundation, where some of my photos and quotes were ultimately featured. She also introduced me to well-connected Parkinson's advocates in the local community. From there, my network began expanding quickly.

I also make a point of reaching out directly to people whose stories resonate with me. Whether I see someone featured on a talk show, read about them online or come across a post in a Facebook group, I often introduce myself and start a conversation.

Facebook groups make this especially easy since you can message people directly. In other cases, it takes a bit more effort to track down an email address, but it's worth it. Many of those profiled in *Living Parkinson's* are people I've connected with through this kind of intentional networking.

I genuinely enjoy talking about my Parkinson's and what I've been able to accomplish despite it. It motivates me. I believe that motivation is rooted in my sense of self-efficacy (see Chapter 1). When you meet others who share a positive mindset, they often enjoy talking about their Parkinson's, too, and for the same reason. It becomes a mutually reinforcing experience.

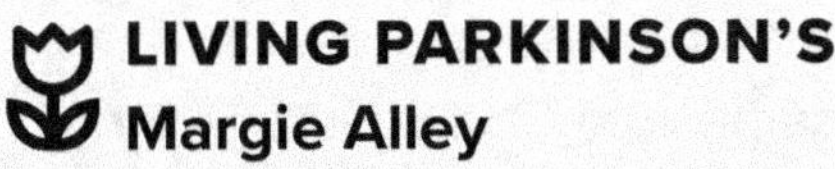

LIVING PARKINSON'S
Margie Alley

PINGPONGPARKINSON WORLD CHAMPION

Margie Alley, a retired social worker and mother, is an athlete and Parkinson's advocate, based in Pleasantville, New York.

Margie was diagnosed in 2013 at age 48. Tennis was her passion—she played in college and continued to play with her friends. It was a big part of her social life. As her Parkinson's symptoms progressed, however, she started experiencing challenges with tennis, particularly freezing of gait. When she would charge the net for a drop shot, her feet would get "glued to the ground" and she would fall onto her knees.

Her bloody knees both shocked and concerned her friends, who were afraid she could get hurt. As she thought about it, they were right—getting hurt would impact her ability to exercise, which is key to managing Parkinson's. As a result, she gradually stopped playing tennis.

Around the time that she was having trouble with her tennis game, a funny thing happened: While at a physical therapy appointment, Margie heard the continuous thumping of loud footsteps overhead and went upstairs to investigate. She discovered a huge ping-pong facility, with tables lined up wall-to-wall. And to her amazement, she saw a sign for a "Parkinson's Ping-Pong Night." Was it fate? She had always enjoyed ping-pong as a kid and just had to check it out. After attending that first gathering, Margie became a regular.

Giving up tennis was difficult, but ping-pong provided an athletic outlet and a new community that was more manageable with her Parkinson's symptoms. Over time, she became more involved, making friends with both Parkinson's patients and volunteers.

Margie described the club interactions as organic. "I would talk to people. And it didn't feel forced. It was very natural—between points or games we would discuss 'Do you have this symptom?' or 'Does this ever happen to you?' It was comfortable. I had tried other support groups that didn't feel as comfortable."

In 2019, the founders of the group organized the first ever PingPongParkinson World Championship—and Margie won the women's gold medal. She has since attended all five championships (held around the world) and recently added another gold medal to her trophy case in the mixed doubles division.

Margie also joined a local women's group. These younger women with Parkinson's share a positive, no-limits attitude, creating a strong connection. Humor is very important to them. When they attended the 2023 World Parkinson's Congress in Barcelona, they unofficially labeled themselves as the "Barcelona Babes," wreaking their own form of havoc while engaging with the Parkinson's community.

These social groups provide friendship and camaraderie in a judgment-free environment that enables Margie to feel comfortable and supported as she and her friends all battle Parkinson's together. "No one likes to be alone on a journey, especially if it's a difficult one," she says. "You want support, you want company. With others with Parkinson's, I can truly be myself. There's no judgment there."

THE POWER OF A STRONG SUPPORT SYSTEM

There are a wide range of benefits you can receive from carefully building your support team:

YOUR CARE TEAM

Coordinated Care	Address motor and non-motor symptoms together
Expert Insight	Provide tailored treatments, therapy, ongoing guidance
Proactive Management	Ensure early intervention before symptoms escalate
Access to Research	Learn about clinical trials and new treatments

FAMILY AND FRIENDS

Emotional Support	Offer empathy, understanding, consistent reassurance
Encouragement	Help you stay on track with treatment and mindset
Purpose	Fuel your commitment and elevate your quality of life
Connection	Reduce loneliness and isolation by staying socially engaged

FELLOW PARKINSON'S WARRIORS

Peer Wisdom	Insights from others navigating Parkinson's day-to-day
Shared Experiences	Provide solidarity through community and connection
Expanded Network	Foster introductions to advocates, resources and new ideas
Confidence Boost	Reap the benefits of inspiration from others who "get it"

Conclusion

Parkinson's is a battle no one should fight alone. Assembling a strong, personalized support system—your care team, your circle of family and friends and your community of fellow Parkinson's warriors—builds a resilient foundation that strengthens every part of the journey. The support you build isn't just emotional, it's strategic. With your team established, you're equipped to win the battle.

Looking Ahead: Strategy #4 – Fight

Now that your support system is in place, you're ready to take action! In the next chapter, we'll talk about how exercise has the potential to slow progression—and how to make it a cornerstone of your battle plan.

TAKEAWAYS/ACTION PLAN

CHAPTER 4

FIGHT

Make Exercise Your Medicine

You need to keep moving. Because
Parkinson's wins if you don't.

WHAT YOU'LL LEARN IN THIS CHAPTER

- ▶ Why exercise is a potential tool to slow
  Parkinson's progression

- ▶ What makes an effective exercise plan

- ▶ How to build a personal program that fits
  your lifestyle

- ▶ How much, how often and how intense—
  backed by science

- ▶ How to use short-term goals to stay motivated
  for the long term

If you were offered a pill to slow your Parkinson's progression, would you take it regardless of the price? Well, our prescription is *exercise*. It's free, but you pay for it with your effort and determination. According to multiple studies summarized by the Parkinson's Foundation, exercise remains the *only* intervention with the potential to slow Parkinson's progression, not just treat symptoms. It needs to be the foundation of your plan.

The specific exercises you do—or whether you do them alone or in a class—are less important than the fact that you're *doing them*. To slow the progression, you need to get moving. And the more intense your movements are, the better.

BUILDING MY EXERCISE PRESCRIPTION

Whenever I encounter a challenge, I return to my problem-solving roots: I learn as much as I can about the problem, evaluate options and build a solution. I approached my exercise-based prescription for Parkinson's the same way.

It began in 2022, when I learned about the exercise regimen that was recommended to impact progression through the Pre-Active PD program (discussed in Chapter 1). My approach included high-intensity aerobic exercise combined with resistance, flexibility and balance components, with (at least) 150 minutes per week as my goal.

Once I understood the requirements, I needed to design a goal-oriented structure that would be both motivating and easy for me to stick with over the long term. The solution? Using athletic events as goals and my training program as the prescription.

I've always been a weekend warrior, enjoying sports and taking part in my share of triathlons and 5K races. But I don't consider myself to be a good athlete. I have always had to work harder than most of my friends—who are more natural athletes—to even come close to competing at their level.

My accomplishments before Parkinson's typically involved finishing in the 75th percentile (meaning behind 75% of the competitors) in these events. I can't count the number of times I finished behind someone 20 years older than me in a triathlon—while watching others already walking their bikes back to their cars, preparing to leave. And that was back when I was much younger! But despite my lack of elite athleticism, I built a plan using events as near-term motivational goals.

FROM DIAGNOSIS TO DETERMINATION

Three years after my diagnosis, after my proactive attitude and self-efficacy had sparked, I took a big leap: I signed up for a triathlon and relay race with my daughter Melissa and for my first-ever Spartan (an obstacle course race) with my oldest son Zack.

While I had done triathlons before, this would be my first endurance race with Parkinson's. I didn't expect the Central Park Relay in NYC to be too taxing (although there was a three-quarter-mile row in Central Park Lake), but this would be my first-ever Spartan—a Spartan Stadion race at Fenway Park in Boston. I had no idea what to expect, either from that event or from my Parkinson's.

A Spartan race combines running with obstacles: crawling under barbed wire, climbing ropes, carrying heavy objects (like buckets of rocks, sandbags or a 100-pound stone), throwing a spear, submerging in a muddy water pit or even jumping over fire. The Stadion is a modified Spartan held at a sports stadium. It would be as much a mental challenge as it would be a physical one. And once I signed up, I wasn't going to back out!

As fall approached, I focused my training on swimming, biking and running for the triathlon. I found a friend in town with a lake house and a rowboat to practice rowing (without spinning in circles). And I joined a CrossFit-style gym to focus on the Spartan.

I had a particularly difficult time with the monkey bars, not necessarily due to a lack of strength but because of the rigidity I had in my left hand from Parkinson's. I was unsure what other surprises my Parkinson's might throw at me during these events—but I was going to find out.

It would be a whirlwind three months, but in the end, it was all worth it. I finished the triathlon only a minute slower than I had nine years earlier, with Melissa cheering me on. We finished the Central Park Relay despite the near-record low temperatures. I can't tell you how cold it was riding a bike—at times over 20 miles per hour—on a brisk 45-degree morning! And rowing the boat together with Melissa, while not a thing of beauty, was a great bonding experience.

The Spartan Stadion with Zack was an adventure: pushups in the Boston Red Sox dugout, a run on the warning track in front of the Green Monster and photos in front of the scoreboard in left field (see below). Finishing to the cheers from my wife and son's girlfriend echoing across the stadium was gratifying. It worked! My experiment with using events as motivation was a complete success. I was in the best shape of my life, I felt terrific about my accomplishments, I had created lasting memories with my kids—all while keeping my Parkinson's at bay. I couldn't ask for more.

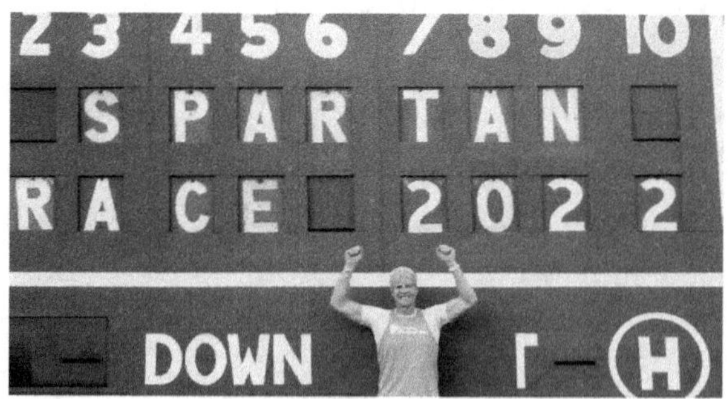

Fenway Park Spartan Stadion

As 2023 arrived, I was ready to build on my recent successes and ratchet up an event-based approach to my exercise program, so I expanded my search to find new and different events to challenge myself. I've continued to build on that formula—today, I seek out an athletic event every couple of months, including Spartans and other obstacle course races, triathlons and even stair climb races. (Yes, they have stair climbs, usually in iconic buildings in big cities. I've raced up the Empire State Building's 1,576 steps in just over 22 minutes.)

Since those first events in 2022, I've finished seven triathlons, ten obstacle course races (Spartans), three Empire State Building stair climbs and various other challenges. But my Parkinson's is always there with me in different ways—I consistently struggle on the monkey bars and similar obstacles due to rigidity in my hands.

These events did more than just improve my fitness, they also created powerful emotional anchors that reinforced my commitment and reminded me why the fight is worth it.

What You Can Do: Set Your First Goal

Choose one physical goal this week that challenges you but is achievable. Write it down and commit to a specific time to complete it (e.g., walk one mile on Saturday morning). Then take the time to celebrate when you complete it! Success will build your confidence and set the foundation for your next goal.

FUELING MOTIVATION WITH "MOMENTS"

I have four adult children, and one or more of them usually participate with me in these events. We've built a library of family memories: hearing my name announced over the loudspeaker as

I cross the finish line in a triathlon with Melissa supporting me … sprinting over the fire jump with Zack, both of us covered in mud, at the end of a Spartan … completing a mud run with Matt on a cold, rainy day … finishing the stair climb on top of the Empire State Building with Jake as we overlook a lit-up Manhattan sky-line on a crisp October evening.

I even miraculously made the podium once in a sprint tri-athlon, coming in third in the 60-to-64 age bracket (although I can't say for sure if there were more than three of us that age in the race that day!).

I participate in these events with my family and friends as *Team Yellen*. As another form of motivation, I designed *Team Yellen* swag: shirts, buffs, sweats and stickers with the hashtags #BeatPD and #NeverGiveUp. We all wear these for motivation.

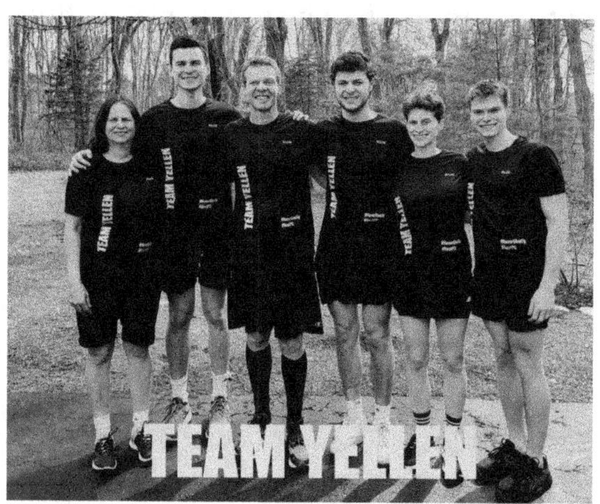

My family in our Team Yellen *attire*

Whether getting dressed in our black *Team Yellen* race attire, crossing the finish line together in our matching outfits or just taking photos together after the race (sometimes covered in mud), it's incredibly gratifying. Just wearing our swag to the gym for a normal workout is motivating for me.

What You Can Do: Motivate Yourself
Pick one way to boost your motivation: Join a class,
wear a team shirt or post a workout photo. Make it fun!
Your fight is personal, but you don't have to do it alone.

FACING CHALLENGES, FINISHING STRONG

In these obstacle course races and other events, practically everyone I see running alongside me looks like they're half my age or younger. This is both challenging and motivating—I take tremendous pride in the fact that there aren't many 60-plus-year-olds competing in these events. And it's probably fair to assume that I'm the only 60-plus-year-old with Parkinson's in most if not all of them.

I use that as motivation when I get tired or am struggling with an obstacle. No matter how exhausted I am at the finish, I always remember that by completing the event, I'm winning another battle in my war with Parkinson's. At the finish of a recent Spartan, race officials were offering a "Spartan Extra Mile" pin to anyone who wanted to run an extra mile. Of course, I couldn't refuse another chance to "stick it" to my Parkinson's.

I wish I could say it is always easy, but it's not. During these races, when I get tired or encounter challenges like a sore knee, I think about my battle and that I can't afford to relent even an inch. I remind myself that it's the amount of heart you possess and your perseverance that enable you to keep going and never quit.

At the end of the day, it's such a good feeling to know I fought through the pain, overcame the doubt and finished strong. Nothing provides more self-confidence and motivation than achieving the goals you set for yourself to fight Parkinson's, plain and simple.

In any race, my goal is always to "finish strong," not to win or make the podium. I've become pretty good at knowing my limits and setting stretch-but-achievable goals. So far, I've been able to succeed in every one of these events (in my own mind, at least)—even at a Spartan where I lost my grip because of the extreme heat, slid down the rope climb and tore the skin off a couple of my fingers.

I remember it well. The Spartan was in Austin, Texas, in May 2024, and it was a 90-plus-degree day. After a few hours in the direct sun, I could feel it—the heat had finally gotten to me. More than halfway up the rope climb, I realized that for the first time, I wasn't going to make it to the top. I lost my grip and slid down the rope. I had to skip a few obstacles that involved climbing or gripping ropes given the state of my fingers. But I tackled the rest of the obstacles and finished the race, bandaged up and in some pain. It really felt good to keep moving and to finish what I had started! And in a couple of weeks, I was back to my normal workout regimen and on to my next event.

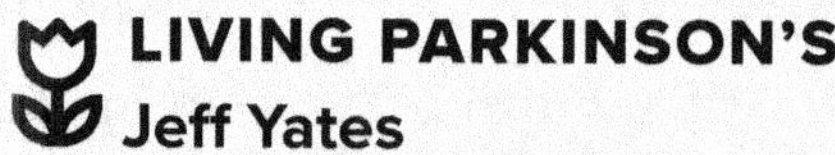 **LIVING PARKINSON'S**
Jeff Yates

FROM BARELY WALKING TO TRIATHLONS

Jeff Yates, psychotherapist, software engineer and dad, is based in London, United Kingdom.

On December 9, 2022, Jeff was thrilled to learn that his wife was pregnant with their first child. Three days later, he went to the doctor with a frozen shoulder and a limp and was told he had Parkinson's. Talk about the highest of highs to the lowest of lows! During the next months, he dealt with various back, leg and arm issues and required a cane to walk. By the time his son was born, he was in a self-proclaimed "dreadful state" and couldn't even pick up his son. He envisioned a future where he wouldn't be able to play football (soccer) with him. That was Jeff's spark: At that moment, everything changed. He looked into the mirror and realized this was going to be up to him.

He joined a local CrossFit gym. "The first couple of months were terrible," he recalls. "I was in a lot of pain and was ready to quit. Then I began taking medication, which enabled me to work out almost every day. That was my goal. I became a new person."

Jeff attributes his success to his "take-charge" attitude and support from his wife and gym instructor. His quality of life, mood, energy and sleep all improved. By early 2024, Jeff was exercising regularly but still couldn't run, swim or ride a bike for more than ten minutes. Over time, though, his routine grew. It included stretching every morning; taking CrossFit classes for strength; running, biking and swimming for cardio; and doing hot yoga. "When it comes to training," Jeff says, "I like to mix it up because I get bored easily. And I enjoyed CrossFit for the social aspect. It wasn't about how much you could lift, but about supporting each other."

As Jeff's condition continued to improve, he was able to start running. It felt amazing. And he signed up for a triathlon just a week after his first run! He completed that first triathlon in September 2024, only a year after he had been walking with a stick (cane), finishing first in his age group. Jeff recalls, "That was one of the best days of my life. My family and friends were there to support me, and my boy was there with a little plastic trophy for me when I finished."

He's become an advocate for exercise, frequently speaking at events on the topic. "It's amazing. You can go from struggling to just walk to running a triathlon," he points out. "It shows what a positive mental attitude can do. It comes down to who you surround yourself with and what you know about your Parkinson's."

Jeff competed in his second triathlon in 2025, with his two brothers joining in to support him.

REWARDING THE FIGHT: MY "WALL OF FAME"

I get a boost from the medals (and other swag) given out to finishers, which I hang on a personal "Wall of Fame" in my home gym. After a race, it's almost ceremonial for me to hang my medal and race number on the Wall and to step back and take stock of what I've accomplished.

It's a daily motivator as I prepare for the next event—a constant reminder that there can't be any quit in my personal battle. Whether it's a certificate for finishing a class or just a photo that has meaning to you, these kinds of "trophies" are another great source of motivation.

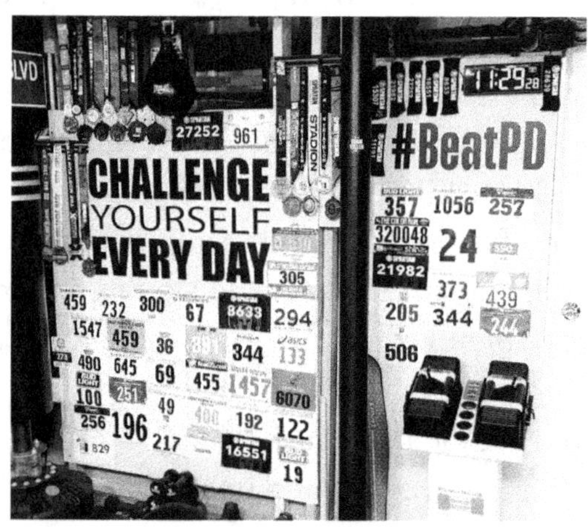

The Wall of Fame in my basement home gym

As I write this book, I'm planning to challenge myself with more events than I did in previous years. Doing more as I get older gives me the confidence that Parkinson's isn't gaining on me. More importantly, these personal challenges keep me focused on my objective and enable me to stick to my Parkinson's "exercise prescription." They also build my self-efficacy, providing both a sense of accomplishment and a motivational boost with each goal I achieve. I encourage you to plan your goals in a way that builds your own self-efficacy.

USING GOALS TO STAY MOTIVATED

I have a somewhat obsessive personality (can you tell?). It contributes to the short-term, goal-oriented approach of self-efficacy. Once I set a goal, I'm fixated on attaining it. I meticulously plan my year of events, continually looking for new options, and once I commit to a specific event, I'm obsessed with completing it. Backing out, in my mind, would be "giving in" and reneging on my commitment.

My family sometimes teases me as I plan far in advance and then stay completely fixated on the goals I set for myself. When I text my kids asking if anyone wants to sign up for an event six months out, I either hear crickets or sarcastic responses—but it's all in jest and I know they have my back. I use my obsessiveness to my advantage: I harness it to keep motivated, stay focused on my exercise regimen and build on my self-efficacy.

> **Every event I complete renews my confidence that I'm managing my Parkinson's progression and gives me a motivational boost to sign up for the next one.**

Every event I compete renews my confidence that I'm managing my Parkinson's progression and gives me a motivational boost to sign up for the next one. It also gives me confidence that I can accomplish anything I put my mind and heart into. My friends and family provide the encouragement and emotional support I need to never let up. This is my winning formula, and a version of it can be yours, too.

MY MEDIEVAL HOME GYM

During COVID, I built a home gym in the unfinished furnace room of my basement (see next page). It's made up mostly of equipment I've collected over the years or inherited from friends and family.

A contractor who came to repair the furnace said, "Wow, this gym is medieval!" I took that as a compliment and a testament to the gym being a no-frills, down-and-dirty place to work out. That was before a few minor upgrades.

Over the years, I cleaned up the concrete walls, put down some old carpets and painted all the ducts and columns black to make it feel more like a gym. I also added mirrors and mounted an old TV, creating a spot for doing YouTube yoga classes, and I put up some of the better photos I have from events and peppered the gym with motivational decals: *#BeatPD*, *No Excuses* and *Never Give Up*, to name a few. Looking for creative ways to upgrade the gym to make it more motivating has become an ongoing hobby of mine. It's a bit less "medieval" now.

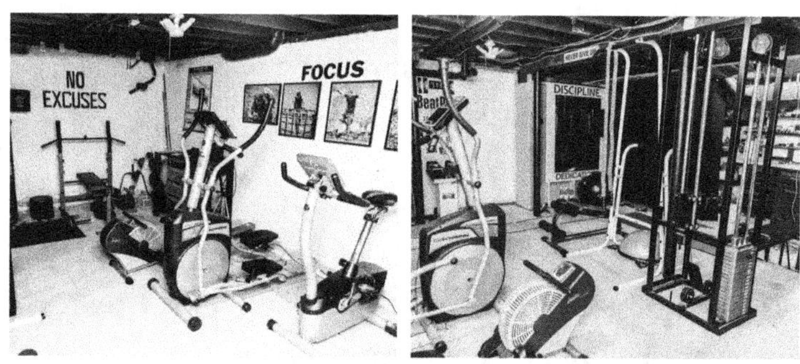

My Basement Home Gym

THE SCIENCE BEHIND THE PRESCRIPTION

In my battle with Parkinson's, I'm always looking for an edge—something that research has proven to be effective. With exercise, I found it. Research supports the benefits of exercise for individuals with Parkinson's, highlighting improvements in motor function, potential neuroprotective effects and enhanced quality of life. Here are a couple of studies I've found:

- ► A Yale University study demonstrated that six months of high-intensity aerobic exercise preserved and even enhanced dopamine-producing neurons in the brain, suggesting a potential slowing of disease progression.[8]

▸ A study analyzing the Rock Steady Boxing® program, which adapts boxing techniques for Parkinson's patients, found significant improvements in satisfaction and quality of life.[9]

The first study above is from Dr. Sule Tinaz of Yale University, who observes:

"The medications we have available are only for symptomatic treatment. They do not change the disease course. But exercise seems to go one step beyond and protect the brain at the neuronal level."[8]

💡 EXPERT INSIGHT
Sule Tinaz on Exercise

Dr. Sule Tinaz, MD, PhD, is a neurologist specializing in movement disorders at Yale Medicine. Her research has been instrumental in demonstrating that exercise can slow the progression of Parkinson's disease.

Q: How can exercise play a role in managing Parkinson's?

DR. TINAZ: Research has shown that exercise can improve symptoms in Parkinson's. Specifically, high-intensity exercise has the potential to slow disease progression and may have neuroprotective effects. Exercise also may reduce mortality and reduce the risk of developing Parkinson's. But more research is needed to firmly establish the disease-modifying and neuroprotective effects of exercise.

Q: Where can people learn more about what exercises are best for them?

DR. TINAZ: The Parkinson's Foundation, in collaboration with the American College of Sports Medicine, recently updated their exercise guidelines for people with Parkinson's. They've posted the most recent information on their website.

Q: How intensely and how often should someone exercise to have the maximum effect?

DR. TINAZ: The focus has been on high-intensity exercise three times a week. We need more research to determine whether moderate-intensity exercise performed more frequently can be equally effective in slowing disease progression and providing neuroprotection.

Q: What advice do you have for individuals who don't currently exercise?

DR. TINAZ: Safety is always the number-one priority. People should consult with their healthcare providers before starting an intense exercise regimen. People who are new to exercise should start slowly, and gradually increase the intensity and frequency of exercise as they build up their stamina. It would be safer to work with a professional like a physical therapist or trainer to come up with a good and sustainable plan, especially in the beginning.

Research Sources from Dr. Tinaz:

Ernst M, Folkerts AK, Gollan R, Lieker E, Caro-Valenzuela J, Adams A, Cryns N, Monsef I, Dresen A, Roheger M, Eggers C, Skoetz N, Kalbe E. Physical exercise for people with Parkinson's disease: a systematic review and network meta-analysis. Cochrane Database Syst Rev. 2024 Apr 8;4(4).

Schenkman M, Moore CG, Kohrt WM, Hall DA, Delitto A, Comella CL, et al. Effect of High-Intensity Treadmill Exercise on Motor Symptoms in Patients With De Novo Parkinson Disease: A Phase 2 Randomized Clinical Trial. JAMA Neurol. 2018 Feb 1;75(2):219-226.

van der Kolk NM, de Vries NM, Kessels RPC, Joosten H, Zwinderman AH, Post B, et al. Effectiveness of home-based and remotely supervised aerobic exercise in Parkinson's disease: a double-blind, randomised controlled trial. Lancet Neurol. 2019 Nov;18(11):998-1008.

de Laat B, Hoye J, Stanley G, Hespeler M, Ligi J, Mohan V, Wooten DW, Zhang X, Nguyen TD, Key J, Colonna G, Huang Y, Nabulsi N, Patel A, Matuskey D, Morris ED, Tinaz S. Intense exercise increases dopamine transporter and neuromelanin concentrations in the substantia nigra in Parkinson's disease. NPJ Parkinsons Dis. 2024 Feb 9;10(1):34.

Yoon SY, Suh JH, Yang SN, Han K, Kim YW. Association of Physical Activity, Including Amount and Maintenance, With All-Cause Mortality in Parkinson Disease. JAMA Neurol. 2021 Dec 1;78(12):1446-1453.

Fang X, Han D, Cheng Q, Zhang P, Zhao C, Min J, et al. Association of Levels of Physical Activity With Risk of Parkinson Disease: A Systematic Review and Meta-analysis. JAMA Netw Open. 2018 Sep 7;1(5):e182421.

RECOMMENDED TYPES OF EXERCISE

Exercise comes in so many forms. Without knowing what works, it can seem overwhelming to determine what to include in your program. While any movement is a good thing, there are some areas that most experts agree you should focus on to slow the progression of your Parkinson's. The American College of Sports Medicine® and the Parkinson's Foundation recommend that exercise programs for people with Parkinson's should include these four key components:

EXERCISE	BENEFITS	EXAMPLES
Aerobic Activity	Boosts endurance and oxygen flow; may slow progression	Brisk walking, cycling, dancing, interval training
Strength Training	Builds muscle, improves posture and bone strength	Weightlifting, push-ups, squats, resistance bands
Balance & Agility	Enhances stability and daily movement efficiency	Yoga, tai chi, Pilates, qigong, dance, boxing
Flexibility & Stretching	Reduces stiffness, improves mobility	Dynamic stretching

I average 60 to 90 minutes a day of overall exercise. I include elements of all the above in my personal routine on a weekly basis and am always looking for new options, specifically those pertaining to balance and agility training (sometimes referred to as neuromotor training).

Looking for "exercise hacks" is another hobby of mine and is something you might enjoy. For example, I purchased a reaction ball, which is a small rubber ball about the size of a baseball with flat sides. Throwing this off a wall produces random directional changes and tests my reflexes; it's almost like being a hockey goalie. I use this to work on my hand-eye coordination.

I also bought a boxing reflex ball, which is a small, spongy ball on an elastic string connected to a headband that you wear. You punch the ball away from you and it springs back. It's not the most graceful of activities, but it is another agility-coordination (neuromotor) exercise, which I believe could help me with my Parkinson's.

I'm not always successful with my experiments. My attempt at juggling balls was an official failure, and I can guarantee I won't be graduating to juggling knives or other sharp objects. While my kids could juggle three balls after 15 minutes of practice, I couldn't even juggle two (sad). I hope I never see a research paper linking slower disease progression to successful juggling!

What You Can Do: Start Smart

Talk to your doctor or physical therapist before beginning any new program. Start small, focus on consistency and gradually build intensity. Parkinson's progression may be unpredictable— but effort is your edge.

EXERCISE PROGRAMS AND CLASSES

For many people, exercise classes offer the structure and accountability to ensure they show up regularly and maintain discipline in their fitness routines. In the Parkinson's community, we are lucky to have many organized exercise programs available to us, including Rock Steady Boxing, Dance for PD®, InMotion® and PWR!Moves®, to name a few.

These programs fall into one or more of the exercise categories I discussed earlier and fit the prescription for improving symptoms. Many other exercise programs have been shown to be beneficial. They often incorporate elements of strength, balance, flexibility and aerobic training, all important for managing symptoms. And new programs are being launched all the time.

> **DISCLAIMER**
> You should always consult with your doctor or physical therapist before starting a new exercise routine. Your routine should be personalized based on your age, fitness level and specific symptoms.

EXERCISE BENEFITS IN BUILDING SELF-EFFICACY

Having reviewed the benefits of exercise on symptom management, let's focus on another significant advantage: building self-efficacy. As you know by now, this has been key for me in maintaining my exercise motivation and pace. Here are just some of the ways self-efficacy has helped me in the battle:

EMPOWERING ME TO CONTROL MY DISEASE PROGRESSION: Engaging in physical activity has provided me with an opportunity to take a proactive role. I believe this has been a factor in my slow progression. The fact that exercise has the potential to slow disease progression keeps me motivated to continue at the rate I'm going.

IMPROVING MY OVERALL FITNESS LEVEL: I feel as though I'm in the best shape of my life given my age. This enables me to live with very few restrictions due to Parkinson's. Being in good shape contributes to overall well-being, optimal health as you age and a positive state of mind.

KEEPING A POSITIVE ATTITUDE: I feel better on the days when I exercise. And finishing a tough workout keeps me confident that I'm not losing ground to Parkinson's. The thrill of crossing a triathlon finish line or leaping over a Spartan fire jump energizes me and keeps me committed to my workouts.

PROVIDING SOCIAL CONNECTIONS: Preparing for and participating in events with family and friends as *Team Yellen* is a unique bonding experience. I can't say enough about the once-in-a-lifetime memories I've built with the other *Team Yellen* participants—and the more people I introduce to these events, the more potential *Team Yellen* members I recruit.

YOUR RACE, YOUR RULES

My intention in sharing my goals and workout regimen is to provide examples for you. Everyone's personal plan must be just that: personal. I know others with Parkinson's who compete in marathons and IRONMAN triathlons that are way beyond my ability, but I never let that discourage me. I stay focused on my goals—and I encourage you to do the same.

What You Can Do: Set an Exercise Goal

Choose a personal fitness goal and *do not* compare it to anyone else's. Write down why it matters to *you*! Reread that when you feel discouraged. This is *your* race, *your* rules.

HOW MUCH IS ENOUGH?
THE SCIENCE OF INTENSITY

Since exercise has been shown to improve symptoms and has the potential to slow progression, the next important questions to answer are, "How much exercise do I need to do?" and "How intense should it be?"

The Parkinson's Foundation recommends 150 minutes of moderate-intensity aerobic exercise a week. The frequency and intensity of specific exercises for a person with Parkinson's depend on their stage of the disease, their overall fitness level and their individual goals. However, research suggests the following general guidelines, broken down by type of exercise:

TYPE OF EXERCISE	FREQUENCY
Aerobic Activity	3 days a week (at least 30 minutes a session)
Strength Training	2–3 days a week (at least 30 minutes a session)
Balance & Agility	2–3 days a week
Stretching	2–3 days a week, but daily if possible

That might sound like a lot, but it amounts to fewer than 60 minutes a day. And remember, this is our best prescription for Parkinson's until researchers find another option. If you have questions, I encourage you to consult with a physical therapist or exercise specialist who has experience with Parkinson's. They can help you create a safe and effective plan tailored to your individual needs.

MEASURING EXERTION

When I first heard the recommendation of 150 minutes a week of moderate-intensity exercise, my first thought was, "What exactly does 'moderate' mean?" As I learned more, I encountered the concept of an "activity minute," which sounded interesting to me. It's a measure of the time spent engaging in physical activity that elevates your heart rate, taking intensity into account. The American Heart Association defines activity minutes in terms of:

▶ **MODERATE-INTENSITY EXERCISE (50% TO 70% OF MAX HEART RATE):** Activities like brisk walking, dancing or gardening (1 minute of moderate-intensity exercise = 1 activity minute).

▶ **HIGH-INTENSITY EXERCISE (70% TO 85% OF MAX HEART RATE):** Activities like running, fast cycling or swimming (1 minute of high-intensity exercise = 2 activity minutes).

Max heart rate can be approximated by subtracting your age from 220 (Max Heart Rate = 220 − Age). The Parkinson's Foundation recommends 150 activity minutes per week. I aim for over 200 minutes a week. For comparison, in my toughest Spartan race—where I found myself on a ski mountain in a rainstorm (it was brutal!)—I hit 351 activity minutes during the almost three hours it took to finish the race. It's a memory I'll never forget, for reasons both good and bad. Because of the conditions and terrain, it was dubbed one of the toughest Spartan races ever—making my finish at 59 years old (four years into Parkinson's) even more satisfying.

There are other, less scientific ways of measuring exertion that anyone can do without dealing with measuring heart rate. Take a look at this chart based on information from the Center for Disease Control (CDC):

OTHER WAYS TO MEASURE EXERCISE INTENSITY

	TALK TEST	RELATIVE INTENSITY
Measurement	*Ability to talk or sing*	*Rate intensity from 0 to 10*
Low intensity	Can sing	1 to 4
Moderate intensity	Can talk, can't sing	5 to 6
High intensity	Can only say a few words	7 to 8

Using the Talk Test, you can approximate your intensity by estimating how difficult it would be for you to talk or sing during your workout. I know that when I run hills in my neighborhood, I'm breathing so hard I can't recite the alphabet out loud.

USING TECH TO STAY ACCOUNTABLE

As a data geek, I enjoy using technology to help measure anything I can about my workouts. My Google Fitbit watch does the job incredibly well—it tracks steps, heart rate, activity minutes and more. I've also used a Polar® heart rate strap in the past, which is probably more accurate for measuring heart rate than a watch on your wrist is.

There are many technology options (smartphone apps, smartwatches) that can help track exercise progress and performance. I wouldn't be surprised if you already have this technology, either on your wrist or in your pocket.

In my opinion, some of the best smartwatches and wearables to monitor your workouts and activity levels include Google Fitbit, Apple Watch®, Garmin® watches and the Polar heart rate strap. These wearables have companion smartphone apps. There are also Parkinson's-specific apps designed to motivate and track activity that are tailored for people exercising with the condition.

These wearables and apps can help track exercise consistency, intensity and performance while providing the motivation to stay active. And companies are always adding new functionality and improving accuracy. Wearables and apps also boost self-efficacy by motivating users as they reach their fitness goals, and they can even facilitate friendly competition.

Wearable tech and Parkinson's-specific apps can enhance motivation and adherence to fitness routines through real-time feedback and progress tracking. Happily, these tools are getting better and cheaper every day.

MAKE EXERCISE FUN AND SUSTAINABLE

Let's talk about a different element of a good exercise program that's really important: fun. Your exercise program needs to be more than just challenging, it needs to be something you actually enjoy. For me, exercise has become a hobby. One reason I do some of these crazy obstacle course races is because I get to problem-solve.

A key challenge for me is how to vary specific exercises in my regimen to train for obstacles. Some of the more challenging ones include the spear throw, the sandbag carry, the bucket carry, the sled push-pull and the rope climb. They're so obscure that you don't find equipment at a typical gym to train for them, so I use YouTube to search "training tips for X" or "build your own X" to figure out how I can build, borrow or buy what I need to train.

To practice for the Spartan spear throw, I've made a spear out of a broom handle, tennis ball and duct tape. I bought a rope that I loop over a tree branch in my yard to practice the rope climb. I've carried cinder blocks around my house and built a push-pull sled by adding pipes and straps with handles to an old pallet I found in the basement. It's amazing what you can learn to build on YouTube!

Sometimes I wonder what my neighbors think when they see me looping a rope over a tree branch in my yard, climbing it a few times and then taking it down. Or walking uphill with an orange Home Depot bucket filled with 40 pounds of rocks on my shoulder or a 60-plus-pound fitness workout sandbag on my back. But maybe the most head-scratching activity is when I throw my homemade Spartan spear at a cardboard box perched on top of a couple of cinder blocks in the driveway.

Your exercise program needs to be more than just challenging, it needs to be something you actually enjoy.

I get a lot of enjoyment out of building these obstacle "hacks" and preparing myself for the races. And it works! In Spartan events, the spear throw has one of the highest failure rates of any obstacle, but I have a personal success rate of over 60%.

This hobby of mine—creating home-built solutions for training—is what led me to build my home gym. These examples of the "hacking" solutions were not only motivating (there's that self-efficacy again), but fun. I encourage you to figure out how you can add the element of fun to your overall efforts. It'll make it easier to stick with your regimen and keep your spirits up, and both are important elements of a successful program.

STAYING SAFE WHILE PUSHING LIMITS

One of the biggest concerns I have about my exercise regimen and the event challenges I sign up for is getting hurt and being forced to stop working out for an extended period. It would be incredibly tough for me both mentally and emotionally if I couldn't exercise and felt like Parkinson's was gaining ground on me.

I've gotten pretty good at listening to my body, pushing myself but knowing my limits—and always staying within those limits. I view this as risk management, and it's why I evaluate every event or activity I'm considering in terms of risk vs. reward. If I think

I could get injured by doing an activity, I pass. I've skipped rock scramble hikes with my friends because of this.

As crazy as it seems in terms of some of the obstacle course races I've done, I can assure you that I approach them in a calculated way (Given what you know about me already, I suppose that should come as no surprise). It has worked for me so far, with no serious injuries to date. If you intend to try something new or challenge yourself as you build an exercise program, always keep risk management in mind. Remember, building an exercise regimen that you can stick to over the long haul—and one that's above all safe—is the goal.

What You Can Do: Add an Exercise

Review the four key elements of exercise: aerobic, strength, flexibility and balance. Choose one to focus on this week and add a 10- to 20-minute session to your calendar. Next week, add another. Build your routine—one session at a time—and always consult with your doctor before changing anything.

Conclusion

Exercise is more than just movement—it's your most powerful weapon in the fight against Parkinson's. Every workout completed and every goal met can build your self-efficacy and potentially slow the disease progression. The key is consistency, intensity and purpose. Exercise is our prescription, one that we fill with effort and a refusal to give in.

Looking Ahead: Strategy #5 – Wellness

Being your strongest self takes more than just movement. In the next chapter, we'll explore how optimizing sleep, stress, nutrition and overall well-being creates the foundation to fight Parkinson's and to live your best life.

TAKEAWAYS/ACTION PLAN

CHAPTER 5

WELLNESS

Be Your Best Self

Wellness isn't about doing everything right—it's about doing what gives you the best chance to win.

WHAT YOU'LL LEARN IN THIS CHAPTER

▶ How the "Four Pillars of Wellness" can support your fight against Parkinson's

▶ Ways to improve nutrition, including hydration and supplements

▶ Why quality sleep and stress management are therapeutic tools

▶ How lifestyle choices impact your healthspan

▶ How to build a personalized, sustainable wellness plan

The average person can get by operating at less than their full potential, but to meet the challenge of Parkinson's, you need every advantage you can get: mentally, physically and emotionally. Bas Bloem, MD, PhD, Director, Radboudumc Center of Expertise for Parkinson & Movement Disorders, observes:

"When I face people with Parkinson's in my clinic, the ones doing the best are the ones who adhere to a healthy lifestyle."

To perform at my best, I've adopted a comprehensive wellness strategy that includes optimal nutrition, quality sleep, stress reduction, mindfulness and low-toxicity living. A balanced approach helps me stay focused, energized and better equipped not just to live with Parkinson's, but to beat it.

Because wellness touches so many areas of life, this chapter explores a wide range of strategies, from nutrition and sleep to mindset and toxin reduction. I'll share what's worked for me, where I've made compromises and why each area deserves attention in your own Parkinson's battle plan.

It's worth mentioning that wellness is personal. It's a unique and dynamic journey, not a one-size-fits-all concept. While I'm sharing my own approach here, *your* wellness is *yours* to define. You should always work with your care team before making any changes to your routine.

What Is Wellness?

Wellness isn't about chasing perfection—it's about pursuing mental, physical and emotional balance to be at your best. For me, it's about making consistent, intentional choices that support energy, resilience and clarity of purpose, each and every day.

Right up front, I want to acknowledge the obvious: we are not machines. Even when we know something might help, doing it 100% of the time isn't always realistic or necessary. I've chosen to live by the "85% Rule": achieving 85% of the ideal state is good enough because that optimizes my health, happiness and ability to stick with it. For instance, I know that unsweetened black coffee is the healthiest option, but to me it tastes like motor oil. Removing sweeteners and creamers would take the enjoyment out of my morning ritual, so I compromise and use a small amount of them.

In each area of wellness I talk about below, I'll define what has been the optimum state for me and where I apply the 85% Rule: compromising where the effort it would take to achieve perfection isn't worth the benefit to me. I'll share where I've made other trade-offs and why they've worked for me.

BEFORE PARKINSON'S: MY EVOLVING APPROACH TO WELLNESS

I started focusing on healthy living in my 20s and 30s, mostly just to stay in good shape. I remember doing the seven-day cabbage soup diet with a group of coworkers to lose a few pounds. We lasted three days. And like a lot of others, I got caught up in the low-fat craze of the 1990s. Anyone else remember Snack-Well's cookies?

It wasn't until I turned 40 that wellness became more intentional. Spurred on by my brother-in-law—who was all-in with nutrition—I got motivated. I read books and stayed away from fad diets and did what I thought was best to be as healthy as possible.

Since my Parkinson's diagnosis and learning about the potential environmental causes of it (see the Q&A with Ray Dorsey in Chapter 2), I've ratcheted up both my education and my commitment to overall wellness. It really is ironic—we often don't get serious about what's best for us until we're confronted with our own vulnerability. My personal approach centers on what's been called the "Four Pillars of Wellness."

THE FOUR PILLARS OF WELLNESS

After learning as much as I could about wellness, I broke things down into the four primary areas of focus: exercise, nutrition, sleep and mindfulness (reducing stress). All of those are built on a foundation of low-toxicity living.

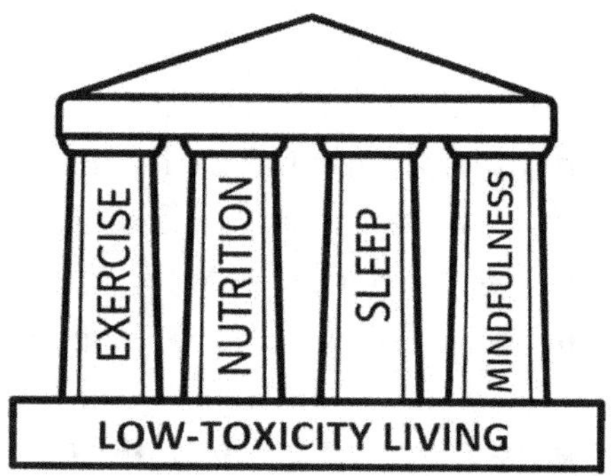

Optimizing and balancing these four pillars has put me in the best position to fight Parkinson's, and I believe they could help you as well.

PILLAR ONE: EXERCISE

Exercise should be a part of everyone's plan, but given its potential benefits for fighting Parkinson's, it's even more important for those of us with the disease to exercise. I've already covered exercise in depth in Chapter 4, so I won't go into it again here. Let me just say that it's perhaps the most important pillar.

PILLAR TWO: NUTRITION – FUELING THE FIGHT

I've found that a brain-healthy diet is remarkably similar to what's recommended for overall health. Most major Parkinson's organizations and medical professionals suggest a balanced, whole-food, plant-focused diet, often aligned with the Mediterranean or MIND diets.[10]

My approach is a modified version of the MIND (Mediterranean-DASH Intervention for Neurodegenerative Delay) diet, which blends the Mediterranean and DASH (Dietary Approaches to Stop Hypertension) diets. I make minor adjustments based on what I've learned that might impact Parkinson's. With nutrition, I follow my No Harm Strategy: If something might help and won't hurt, I'll consider it. For example, I've read mixed evidence about dairy and its potential link to inflammation,[11] so I've cut out most dairy—I replace milk in my coffee with oat or almond creamers.

Here are the nutrition principles I follow ... about 85% of the time:

My Core Nutrition Principles – Foods to Include

FOOD	BENEFIT
Leafy greens & vegetables	Rich in folate, antioxidants and fiber (spinach, kale)
Berries	Support cognitive health (blueberries, strawberries)
Whole grains	Provide steady energy, fiber (oats, quinoa, whole wheat)
Nuts	Support brain and heart health
Legumes	High in fiber and plant-based protein
(Fatty) fish	Rich in omega-3 fatty acids supporting cognitive health
Poultry	Brain-supportive protein source
Olive oil	A cornerstone because of its anti-inflammatory benefit
Hydration & fiber	Helps with Parkinson's-related constipation
Probiotics & prebiotics	Fermented foods support gut health

My Core Nutrition Principles – Foods to Limit or Avoid

FOOD	CONCERN
Red meat	Choose lean cuts to limit saturated fats
Butter & margarine	Substitute with olive oil
Dairy	Can cause inflammation
Cheese	Limit due to saturated fat content
Pastries & sweets	Can cause inflammation and impact gut health
Fried or fast foods	Limit to reduce inflammation and saturated fats
Ultra-processed foods	Foods with many ingredients, preservatives, added sugars
Caffeine & alcohol	Limit to moderate intake

For me, food is a major source of pleasure, not just fuel to satisfy my hunger. Fortunately, I like most of the recommended foods. I'm a big fan of fish (especially sushi), chicken and beans. But I also enjoy a juicy hamburger, a slice of pizza, a toasted bagel and salt added to my food.

I've chosen not to deprive myself of those things—I just eat them in moderation (There's that 85% Rule again). I've also made the personal choice to eliminate most alcohol except for an occasional cold beer on a hot day or a Guinness on tap, which I can't resist.

What You Can Do: Modify Your Diet One Step at a Time

Try to adopt some of the generally accepted recommendations, but don't deprive yourself to the point where it impacts your happiness. That matters, too! Stick to the 85% Rule and try to average that level of commitment across the categories. See which changes make you feel better and stick with them.

I've also explored intermittent fasting, which may support mitochondrial[12] and gut health. While there's no clear consensus on the matter, some evidence suggests that giving your digestive system a 12- to 14-hour rest overnight may be beneficial. And fasting also naturally reduces snacking.

I try to fast for 12-plus hours from dinner to breakfast, but I often succumb to snacking. I rarely go longer than 14 hours without eating anything because I enjoy my coffee in the morning and just don't like it black. And I don't skip late-night dinner parties or deprive myself of any special activities. But on a typical weeknight, an overnight fast is surprisingly doable (and can't hurt).

Hydration: Fuel for Your Body

About two-thirds of our body weight is water—our cells need it to function and we can't survive without it. Staying well-hydrated is an often overlooked but powerful way to support your health. For people with Parkinson's, dehydration can worsen constipation—already a common challenge—as well as impact other symptoms.[13]

Drinking 6 to 8 glasses of water a day is a common target for the general population, though your personal needs may vary based on activity level, medications or environment. Carrying a reusable water bottle (stainless steel is an option as opposed to plastic; see the Low-Toxicity Living section later in this chapter) and sipping throughout the day is one simple habit that can have a real impact on how you feel, move and think.

I drink a 16- to 20-ounce glass of water with my first dose of medication every morning and then do my best to keep myself hydrated throughout the day, especially when I exercise in warm weather. I almost always drink 12-plus ounces of water with every pill, both to stay hydrated and to maximize absorption. I sometimes add a natural, sugar-free flavor enhancer—something like a fruit-infused twist—to mix it up a bit.

What You Can Do: Hydrate with a Twist

If you get bored with plain water as you commit
to staying hydrated, try adding a twist of lemon
or an herbal infusion to add variety.

Supplements: Use with Intention

The topic of supplements can be overwhelming, with conflicting advice and bold claims coming at you from all directions, and I'm definitely not in a position to make recommendations. I know people who take a long list of supplements and some who don't take any. In general, I follow my No Harm Strategy and rely on established Parkinson's and medical sources as guidance. I'm not suggesting anyone take these supplements, but I'm sharing my list in case it's helpful as a reference.

I take vitamin B9 (folate), vitamin B12, vitamin D3, CoQ10 (because I'm on a statin), curcumin, resveratrol, fish oil, magnesium (for restless leg syndrome), creatine and a probiotic (for gut health). They are all focused on general wellness.

Some have shown mixed results in terms of how they impact Parkinson's progression, but none of them would make someone think that I have Parkinson's—many of these were recommended to me before my diagnosis. I take moderate doses (i.e., within the Recommended Dietary Allowance [RDA] if there is one) and review them with my doctor at each appointment.

What You Can Do: Be Careful with Supplements

The industry is unregulated and manufacturers
can make bold claims. Consult with your doctor
before taking any supplements! And if you choose
to use any, try to buy well-established brands or
those tested by third-party labs.

I'm not going to discuss medications or the timing of protein with medications here because any discussions related to medications should be reviewed with your care team. Again, note that what I'm sharing here is my *personal* approach—one that I review with my nutritionist, primary movement disorder specialist and primary care physician at every appointment.

PILLAR THREE: SLEEP – YOUR BODY'S RESET BUTTON

Just as diet fuels the body, sleep gives it a chance to recover, repair and reset. You can eat all the right foods, but if your sleep is poor, your body might not benefit from the nutrients, nor will your brain have the downtime it needs to function well, especially with Parkinson's in the picture.

I try to keep a consistent schedule and aim for at least seven hours each night. I also try to wake up naturally and not to an alarm—that really helps me start the day feeling refreshed. In contrast, waking up "unnaturally" feels like a shock to my system.

I find my sleep pattern to be circadian. I wake up earlier in the summer and later in the winter—but always try to get seven-plus hours of shut-eye. I also find that eating a lighter dinner and starting an intermittent fast in the evening help me sleep better.

For those with Parkinson's, prioritizing sleep is important, as sleep disturbances are common and can exacerbate symptoms. Poor sleep doesn't just make you tired, it can impact both motor and non-motor symptoms.[14]

On the positive side, prioritizing high-quality sleep can make a measurable difference. Even modest changes—such as consistent bedtimes, reducing screen exposure before sleep, avoiding late-night caffeine and keeping a cool, dark sleeping environment—can enhance restorative sleep. Simply put: When you sleep well, your body heals, your mind clears and you're better equipped to fight Parkinson's each day.

What You Can Do: Create a Sleep Schedule

Stick to a consistent sleep schedule, even on weekends (if possible). Create a calming pre-bed routine: Dim the lights, avoid screens for an hour before bed and keep your bedroom cool, dark and quiet. Avoid large meals or alcohol late at night. If racing thoughts keep you up, try relaxation techniques. And wake up to the sunlight to get yourself going.

PILLAR FOUR: MINDFULNESS – REDUCE STRESS, THE INVISIBLE ENEMY

If sleep is your chance to recharge, mindfulness is the conscious effort to prevent the stress of the day from draining your energy and stealing your focus. For people living with Parkinson's, that hidden drain caused by stress isn't just inconvenient, it can intensify both motor and non-motor symptoms.[15] While stress is like a constant friction draining precious energy, mindfulness can be like a pressure relief valve—it's a tool to keep stress at a manageable level.

Over time, I've gained the perspective to know which problems are worth stressing over and which ones just aren't worth the energy. I've always told my kids that no matter how bad things may seem in the moment, most of life's challenges turn out to be manageable.

As I've tried to show by example, even a diagnosis like Parkinson's can be managed to a degree. But given the damaging effects of stress on overall health, I make a conscious effort (and constantly remind myself!) to not let unimportant things bother me.

While I don't meditate as part of my routine, if I feel like my stress level is increasing, I remove myself from the situation, take a breath and do my best to relax. I try to keep in mind that whatever is causing concern will only get worse if I continue to stress over it. If I find that something is sticking with me, I'll use a meditation smartphone app to give myself a 5–10 minute time-out.

Gratitude: A Practice of Mindfulness

Gratitude might be a surprising topic in a Parkinson's book, but appreciating what I have has always been important to me. Practicing gratitude doesn't mean ignoring the challenges of Parkinson's, it means choosing to focus on what's still good.

I often remind myself of everything I have as opposed to the challenges I'm facing. I've found that many other Parkinson's warriors I meet who are doing well share a similar outlook. Gratitude helps shift your mindset from loss to resilience, and over time, that shift can reduce stress and build emotional strength.

Stress and Parkinson's

Stress is more than an emotional state—it's a physiological force that can influence the day-to-day experience of Parkinson's. Research has shown that stress can exacerbate motor symptoms like tremors and freezing of gait as well as non-motor symptoms such as sleep problems and depression.[14]

Fortunately, the flip side has also been shown to be true: Embracing mindfulness to reduce stress can improve both physical and mental functioning. Practices like yoga, tai chi and qigong can reduce stress while filling a component of the recommended exercise program reviewed in Chapter 4. These benefits reinforce a powerful truth: Mindfulness isn't a luxury, it has value as a therapeutic strategy. Whether it's through meditation, movement, journaling, music or simply slowing down, mindfulness isn't just good for reducing stress—it can be part of your prescription.

Some Stress Might Be Positive

Some researchers suggest that exposure to moderate, manageable stress—the kind you can master—can actually make you stronger and more resilient. This isn't the chronic stress that wears you down, but just enough stress to challenge you without overwhelming you. Think of it as a cycle of challenge and recovery. I like to compare it to resistance training: Push too hard, and you risk injury; don't push at all, and you won't grow stronger.

This same principle applies to life with Parkinson's. Facing manageable challenges like exercising, learning something new or setting small goals can build mental and physical resilience. And that can help you stay sharper, stronger and more engaged.

What You Can Do: Create a Stress Relief Plan

You can't eliminate stress, but you *can* control your response to it. If you feel stressed, try building a daily practice that helps you stay calm: deep breathing, meditation, tai chi, qigong or even going for a quiet walk. Apps like Headspace® or Insight Timer® can guide your mindfulness routines. Start small. Even five to ten minutes a day can make a noticeable difference in how you feel—and how you fight.

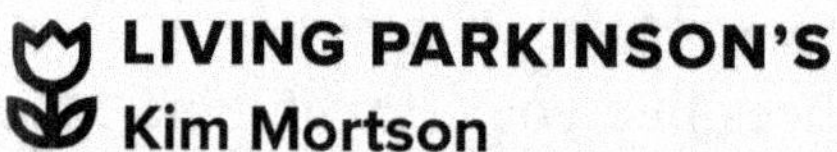 **LIVING PARKINSON'S**
Kim Mortson

FIGHTING PARKINSON'S WITH CALM

Kim Mortson, a certified personal trainer and nutrition coach and founder of Body Design, a yoga and fitness studio, is based in Fenelon Falls, Ontario, Canada.

When Kim Mortson was diagnosed with Parkinson's, it felt like a curveball thrown into an already difficult season of life—she was navigating personal issues and then was suddenly faced with a new challenge. A lifelong personal trainer and movement coach, Kim had spent more than two decades helping others stay strong and active, so when her body began to betray her before the diagnosis, it felt like cruel irony. She had spent her life promoting movement, only to be struck by a disease that was gradually stealing hers.

By the end of 2023, the emotional toll had grown unbearable. "I was at my lowest," she recalls, describing a time when her mobility had seriously deteriorated. "I wasn't just physically weak. I was emotionally broken."

Then something shifted.

It wasn't a specific moment in time. It was a transition: a decision to stop spiraling and start rebuilding. Kim began to see that while she couldn't control Parkinson's, she *could* control how she responded to it. And at the core of her response was stress. "Stress was making everything worse. It impacted both my motor and non-motor symptoms. I had to find a way to let it go—not just once, but every day."

That realization became her turning point. Kim committed herself to managing her internal world as fiercely as she had once trained her physical body. She began journaling, meditating and practicing gratitude. She rewired her thinking to focus on what she *could* do rather than on what she had lost. She returned to gentle movement, rediscovered her voice through advocacy and reconnected with her purpose. Slowly, her energy returned. Her strength returned. So did her spark. Stress hadn't disappeared, but it no longer controlled her.

Today, Kim is thriving, not because her disease has reversed, but because her mindset has. She lives with intention, builds daily routines that support her peace and continues to help others navigate their own battles. Her journey is a living example of what she teaches: that while unmanaged stress can accelerate decline, managed stress can unlock resilience. "Stress is always going to be there," she observes. "But I've learned to meet it differently. I don't let it define my day anymore."

Wellness is now her anchor. From consistent movement and healthy eating to deep breathing and emotional honesty, Kim treats her daily habits like medicine. She listens to her body and her mind—nurturing both with compassion and consistency.

Her message to others is clear: You don't have to pretend you're okay, but you also don't have to stay stuck. Managing stress isn't just a mental health strategy, it's a Parkinson's strategy. "This disease hits hard, but I hit back—with calm."

LOW-TOXICITY LIVING: CLEARING THE PATH

Low-toxicity living is the practice of minimizing exposure to harmful environmental chemicals in your daily life: in your food, water, air, home products and personal care products. The goal is to reduce the overall "toxic burden" on the body so your natural systems can function more efficiently.

It comes down to giving your body the right fuel—healthy food and lots of water—and avoiding harmful substances like cigarettes, too much alcohol, pesticides and other toxic chemicals. It's become important enough to me that I've encouraged my kids to follow suit.

For me, low-toxicity living has involved choosing organic fruits and vegetables, limiting ultra-processed foods, drinking filtered water, filtering the air in my home, using natural personal care products and avoiding harmful chemicals.

For fruits and vegetables, I focus on the Dirty Dozen™ list

published annually by the Environmental Working Group (EWG)[16], buying organic for anything on that list. These are the items most likely to carry pesticide residues, even after washing. There is also a Clean Fifteen™ list, featuring the items that have the lowest amounts of pesticide residues according to EWG's analysis.

EWG also certifies other personal products like sunscreens, moisturizers, shampoos and other personal care products, many of which are available on Amazon. For most of these personal care items, I've switched brands to those on the EWG-approved list.

It comes down to giving your body the right fuel.

In light of growing concerns about plastics—which potentially leach harmful chemicals, especially when exposed to heat—I've made a conscious effort to reduce my use of plastic. One simple change I've made is replacing plastic water bottles and food storage containers with glass and stainless-steel alternatives.

Enabling Your Body to Focus on Parkinson's

Growing evidence links environmental toxins (pesticides, herbicides, heavy metals, certain industrial chemicals) to an increased risk of developing Parkinson's.[17] Several high-profile studies have shown that long-term exposure to substances like trichloroethylene (TCE) can damage the same dopamine-producing neurons that are lost in Parkinson's. These chemicals can enter the body through food, water, air and even personal care products, often accumulating over time and interacting with genetic vulnerabilities.

For people already living with Parkinson's, adopting a lower-toxicity lifestyle isn't about fear; it's about giving their body the cleanest environment possible to function, heal and respond to treatment. Your body already works hard managing Parkinson's. Reducing your exposure to external toxins may help lower inflammation, improve gut health and lighten the stress load on your nervous system, enabling more room for healing and resilience. Simple changes to your food, home and self-care routines can make a meaningful difference.

What You Can Do: Remove One Potentially Toxic Item

Choose organic produce when possible, especially when it comes to fruits and vegetables on the Dirty Dozen list. Avoid chemical-laden cleaning products and opt for natural alternatives. Read labels on personal care products. Use glass or stainless-steel containers instead of plastic, especially when heating food. Every small change can lighten the load on your system and help you fight Parkinson's from a stronger position.

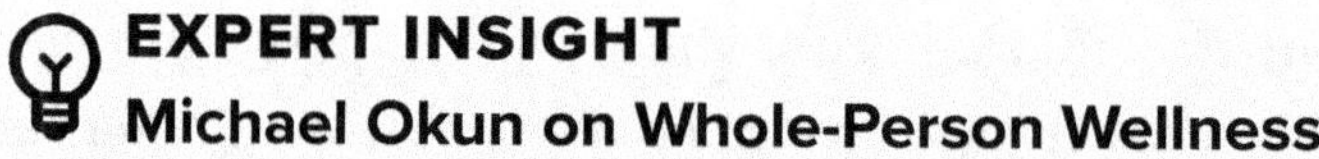

EXPERT INSIGHT
Michael Okun on Whole-Person Wellness

Dr. Michael Okun is Director of the Norman Fixel Institute for Neurological Diseases at the University of Florida and Medical Advisor to the Parkinson's Foundation. He is a leading expert in Parkinson's care and author of 10 Secrets to a Happier Life *and* The Parkinson's Plan.

Q: What role does overall wellness play in managing Parkinson's?

DR. OKUN: Wellness is foundational. Parkinson's is not a death sentence. It's a very livable disease, and the way you approach it can make all the difference. That starts with reframing your mindset. Too many people hear "Parkinson's" and think "Alzheimer's," imagining rapid decline. We need to untangle those assumptions. With the right wellness plan, people can live well for a long time.

Q: You've said exercise can be more powerful than medication. Can you explain?

DR. OKUN: Absolutely. Exercise is like medicine—it's one of the most powerful tools we have. It not only helps control symptoms but also appears to possibly slow disease progression. Everyone should have a personalized exercise plan, ideally developed with a physical therapist. From a wellness standpoint, aiming for 7,500 steps a day seems to hit a sweet spot. And with body composition, maintaining some muscle mass matters—a little extra weight, even five pounds above your "ideal," can actually be beneficial with Parkinson's.

Q: How important are nutrition and supplements?

DR. OKUN: Nutrition is a big part of the wellness equation, though it's highly individualized. A Mediterranean-style diet—rich in vegetables, fruits, whole grains and healthy fats—is generally a good place to start. It's anti-inflammatory and supports brain health. That said, it's important to give yourself room to enjoy food, too. Most people with Parkinson's will also benefit from a simple multivitamin. It's a safe baseline to support general health.

The multivitamin is especially important if you're on dopamine replacement therapy, as it helps replenish key co-factors, reduces the chance of numbness in your feet and lowers homocysteine levels—an important factor linked to dementia and cardiovascular disease. But don't just guess, test! Blood panels can reveal deficiencies and help guide those decisions.

Q: How does sleep tie into wellness for people with Parkinson's?

DR. OKUN: Sleep is critical—and often overlooked. People with Parkinson's tend to have fragmented sleep and are more likely to have sleep apnea. Poor sleep means less cognitive and physical reserve the next day. I recommend using wearable sleep trackers to understand your sleep patterns. The goal is to get six to eight hours of *actual* sleep per night. Good sleep doesn't just feel better, it supports brain health and function.

Q: Stress is a major issue for many people. How can it be managed effectively?

DR. OKUN: Stress is toxic to the brain, especially to areas central to Parkinson's. One of my core rules is to live a life of Zen. That means minimizing unnecessary drama. If someone in your life is constantly stressing you out, maybe it's time to set boundaries. The more Zen you are, the better you'll do.

Q: For someone starting out, what are the most important things they can do?

DR. OKUN: Start with the basics: Protect your environment. Wash your fruits and vegetables. Use a good water filter—especially if you have well water—to reduce exposure to environmental toxins, which may make symptoms worse and increase Parkinson's risk for those around you. Exercise and sleep should also be top priorities: They aren't just good habits, they're essential tools in managing this disease. And we also need to make sure people know Parkinson's is *livable*, but we each need a Parkinson's plan.

HEALTHSPAN: LIVING WELL FOR LONGER

Healthspan is the length of time in your life that you remain healthy, functional and free from serious disease or disability. It's not just about how long you live—that's *life*span—it's about how well you live.

For people with Parkinson's, healthspan is a meaningful goal. While the disease may be chronic and progressive, the focus shifts to maximizing quality of life for as many years as possible: staying active, sharp, independent and emotionally well.

This chapter could have just as easily been titled "Maximizing Healthspan," as many of the examples I give here could help contribute to a longer healthspan. Much of what I've learned about healthspan also aligns with lessons from the world's blue zones: places where people live longer, healthier lives.[18]

EVERYDAY MOVEMENT: LESSONS FROM THE BLUE ZONES

I want to introduce a related topic that I believe in strongly and that merits some discussion: movement. I had been working out one to two hours a day, but because of my job and lifestyle, I used to spend about 10 to 12 hours a day sitting. That made me take a closer look at how much of my day was still sedentary despite the time I spent exercising.

I've long been a follower of Blue Zones® and have tried to incorporate aspects of that lifestyle into my routine (see next page for a deeper dive).

WHAT ARE BLUE ZONES?

Blue zones are regions of the world where people live longer and healthier lives compared to the global average. These areas were identified by Dan Buettner along with a team of scientists and demographers who studied populations with high concentrations of centenarians (people who live to 100 and beyond).

Buettner and his colleagues identified common lifestyle factors that contribute to longevity in these regions, known as the Power 9® principles. These include natural movement, a sense of purpose, stress reduction, plant-based eating, moderate alcohol consumption, faith or spirituality, strong family bonds and social engagement:

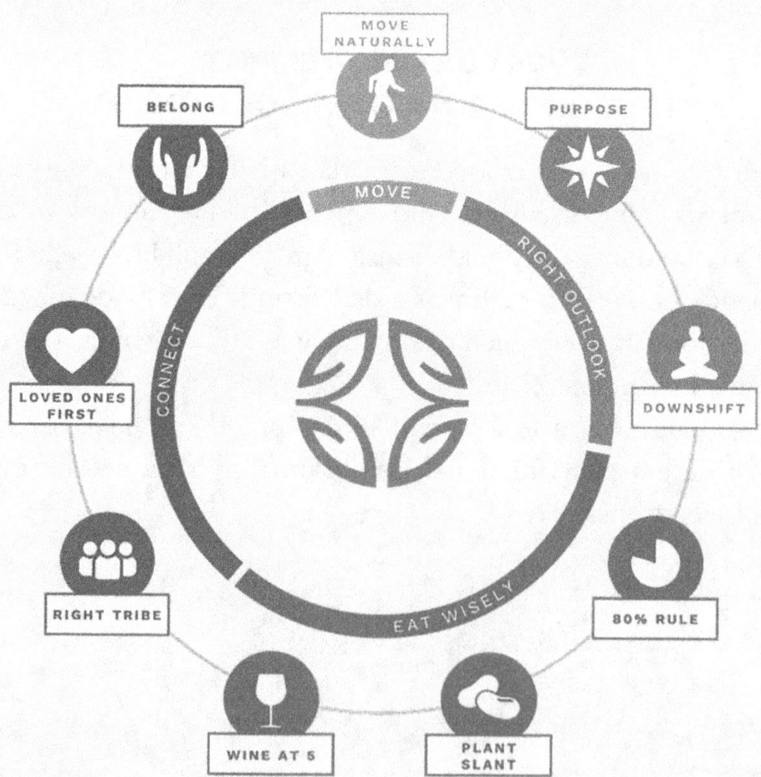

One thing that stands out about blue zone communities is how they incorporate movement into their daily routines—not through gyms or structured workouts, but by simply living in a way that keeps them active throughout the day. That principle really resonated with me and reinforced my commitment to finding more ways to stay in motion beyond just workouts.

Besides daily workouts, I now do whatever I can to avoid being sedentary. I take the stairs instead of elevators or escalators. When parking in a large lot, I opt not to search for the "perfect spot" and instead I park in the first spot I see, even if it means walking farther—though I'll admit, that parking strategy doesn't always make me popular with whoever's in the car with me.

To combine socialization with movement, I take frequent walks with friends. I have a standing two-mile neighborhood walk with a couple of friends every Saturday and Sunday morning when we're free; we stop at a local business for a coffee along the way.

I also started working at a standing desk and taking hourly breaks between work meetings to walk up and down a flight of stairs. These small changes add up. A therapist once suggested this routine to help with minor back pain, and it's been a game changer.

Blue zones offer us a lot of great tips for healthy living. While they're not necessarily Parkinson's-related, incorporating these ideas into our lives can absolutely support our fight to live well with the disease.

What You Can Do: Take Movement Breaks

Look for opportunities to add natural movement to your day: think taking the stairs instead of elevators, walking to meetings or even doing more household chores. Limit long periods of sitting by standing up or stretching every hour. Even a short walk around the house can help.

EASTERN MEDICINE: KEEPING AN OPEN MIND

I've read several books and personal stories from individuals who credit disciplines like qigong or acupuncture with improving their Parkinson's symptoms. Personally, I rely on Western medicine as the foundation of my care.

But I also recognize that Western medicine doesn't have all the answers and that what seems unexplainable today may be better understood by science in the future. After all, many treatments we now take for granted would have been considered mystical a century ago.

That's why I believe each person should evaluate these approaches for themselves. If a therapy is safe, aligns with your values and offers potential benefit, it may be worth exploring—as long as it complements rather than replaces evidence-based care.

I've investigated a few Eastern-based options, including trying acupuncture, and I've added a ten-minute qigong session to my routine twice a week. I find qigong helps "loosen me up," so to speak, and relieves tightness in my lower back, especially in the morning.

Some results attributed to Eastern practices may eventually find scientific validation. I choose to stay open-minded—and I invite others to explore these paths thoughtfully, with safety and guidance from their care team.

KEEPING MENTALLY SHARP: TRAIN YOUR BRAIN

While Parkinson's is often defined by its physical symptoms, the non-motor effects (insomnia, digestive issues, softened speech, loss of smell, etc.) can be just as significant. That's why staying mentally sharp is a core part of my wellness plan. Parkinson's can affect memory, attention and executive function, but there's evidence that staying mentally active can help slow cognitive decline and promote brain resilience.

For me, that means making mental engagement a daily habit, not as a chore, but as something integrated into how I work, relax and enjoy life. I currently work 40-plus hours a week, and I consider that in itself a major form of mental training: For me, working entails problem-solving, decision-making, writing and collaborating.

Beyond work, I still make time for other forms of stimulation that exercise different parts of my brain. I aim to spend time every day doing a mix of activities: solving puzzles, playing strategic games, watching documentaries and practicing mindfulness.

The key is variety and sustainability—I choose things that are both mentally challenging and personally enjoyable. Whether it's solving a crossword or fixing a broken household item, I see it as exercise for my brain. But it's also wise to change things up and try something new, like working on a different type of puzzle or even learning an instrument.

The act of writing this book has been a huge challenge for me—it has pushed me to do something completely out of my comfort zone. Just like working out keeps your body strong, keeping your mind engaged builds mental resilience.

What You Can Do: Find One Game or Puzzle That Challenges You

Keep your brain in the game! Choose mentally engaging activities you enjoy and do them regularly. Reading, writing, puzzles, music, games or learning a new skill all count. Think of doing those things as exercising your brain. The more you use it, the more you protect it.

RECENT RESEARCH SUPPORTING THE POWER OF WELLNESS

An article appearing in *The Lancet Neurology* (October 15, 2025 Online Edition) reinforces the power of wellness in the Parkinson's battle: "The role of lifestyle interventions in symptom management and disease modification in Parkinson's disease" describes the emerging evidence that increasing physical activity, adopting healthy dietary patterns and managing stress can all provide symptomatic benefits and potentially slow neurodegeneration in Parkinson's disease.[19]

Conclusion

Wellness isn't about perfection, it's about putting yourself in the best position every day to fight back. You don't need perfection—you just need to make consistent, intentional choices. Each step toward better wellness builds your strength to push back! Every act of wellness you take helps you feel stronger, think more clearly and live more fully.

You won't always control your symptoms, but you *can* control the environment you create for your body and mind. Wellness is how you tilt the odds in your favor. It's not a side strategy—it's part of your battle plan.

Looking Ahead: Strategy #6 – Advocacy

When you take care of yourself, you gain the clarity and confidence to not only optimize your *own* journey but to help others on theirs. In the next chapter, we'll explore how to turn your experience into action, whether it's raising awareness, influencing policy or simply speaking up. Advocacy isn't about being loud—it's about being heard.

TAKEAWAYS/ACTION PLAN

CHAPTER 6

ADVOCACY

Make Your Voice Heard

Change often begins with a single voice that refuses to stay silent.

WHAT YOU'LL LEARN IN THIS CHAPTER

▶ Why advocacy matters and how it can drive change

▶ How to get started, from local events to national policy initiatives

▶ The many forms advocacy can take

▶ The personal benefits of advocacy: renewed purpose and a sense of empowerment

▶ Real stories of impact that prove one voice makes a difference

Advocacy is the act of amplifying your voice and turning your experiences into action. It's how individuals with Parkinson's make a difference: influencing research, improving care, inspiring legislation and accelerating the search for a cure. It's a way to take charge not just of your own journey, but of the collective journey we all share.

You don't need political experience to make an impact. You just need your story—and the willingness to share it.

MY JOURNEY TOWARD ADVOCACY

Advocacy usually isn't the first thing that comes to mind after a Parkinson's diagnosis. Most of us—myself included—start by focusing inward, trying to make sense of what the diagnosis means and how to manage it. That's natural.

At the outset, I focused on what my diagnosis meant for me and my family; the world around me kind of faded into the background. That period lasted about three years. But eventually, it began to shift. I began to look beyond my own experience and think about the bigger picture. What could I do to contribute? How could I support the broader Parkinson's community?

I had never thought about advocacy and didn't know much about it. I hadn't realized that simply telling my story could spark change. Advocacy began for me not with a plan, but with the realization that my voice could count for more than just me.

Living Parkinson's isn't only about helping yourself. It's about being part of something bigger—shaping a better future for everyone facing this disease. That's where advocacy comes in.

Still, the idea of advocacy can feel intimidating. For some, it's the fear of public speaking, which is often ranked as one of the most common fears. For others, it's the vulnerability of sharing something so personal—or the worry about visibly experiencing symptoms while doing it, since anxiety tends to intensify them. These are real challenges that are part of the decision we all have to make when considering being an advocate.

But those weren't my specific hesitations—mine was going public online.

GOING PUBLIC: A PERSONAL DECISION

I've embraced many forms of advocacy over the years, presenting at events or sharing my story in person. But there's one boundary I held for a long time: I chose not to go public with my diagnosis online. Not because I was ashamed, but because I understood the permanence of digital visibility—once something is put online, it's out there forever. So, even while being active and vocal in the community, I've tried to keep my diagnosis off the internet.

But now, more than six years after my diagnosis—and at age 62—I've reached a point where the rewards of going fully public outweigh my concerns. With the launch of *Living Parkinson's*, my story will be both in print and online. The website (livingparkinsons.com) will be live, and I'll be posting content through @LivingParkinsons on Instagram.

I'm sharing all this for a couple of reasons. First, I don't want anyone reading this to think my decision to hold off on going online was due to any embarrassment about being a person with Parkinson's. I take pride in what I've accomplished and am honored to be an advocate for the community. Second, it's to underscore that every person makes these types of decisions for their own reasons and on their own schedule. There's no right or wrong timeline. As the saying goes, until you've walked a mile in someone else's shoes, you can't truly understand their path.

I was able to begin my advocacy without going public when I learned about the National Plan to End Parkinson's.

MY VOICE IN ACTION:
THE NATIONAL PLAN TO END PARKINSON'S

In August 2022, I attended a webinar hosted by The Michael J. Fox Foundation. The topic was the National Plan to End Parkinson's Act—bipartisan legislation aimed at creating a coordinated national response to the disease. It was the first I'd heard of it.

> The **NATIONAL PLAN TO END PARKINSON'S ACT** is the first-ever federal legislation focused solely on preventing, treating and ultimately curing Parkinson's disease. The plan creates a coordinated national strategy across federal agencies, such as the National Institute of Health (NIH), Centers for Disease Control (CDC) and the Environmental Protection Agency (EPA), all led by the Department of Health and Human Services (HHS) to accelerate research, improve care and address potential environmental and genetic causes.

The webinar was a call to action to urge local representatives to move the bill forward. The Foundation suggested we join them on calls with our representatives to gain support for the National Plan. Although I'd never spoken with anyone in government before, this was an easy sell for me—I enjoyed telling my story and already had significant professional experience both with public speaking and as a company spokesperson. I saw the calls as a perfect opportunity to make a difference, and I was immediately on board. This would be self-efficacy at its finest: a short-term goal to get a sponsorship commitment that directly supported my objective (see Chapter 1).

The calls were coordinated and led by the associate director of public policy at the Foundation. She scheduled a 30-minute video call with the legislative aide covering healthcare for each

Connecticut representative. We met with aides of Representative Jim Himes (D-CT) and Senator Richard Blumenthal (D-CT). We prepped for the call and agreed on the flow and my message. My message focused on two key points:

1. My success in managing Parkinson's to date was largely due to the knowledge I'd gained on my own—and more people with the disease deserved access to the same information in a structured manner.

2. A coordinated national effort was essential. Agencies like the EPA and CDC needed to communicate and work together if we were serious about ending Parkinson's.

The calls went very smoothly and took about 15 minutes. The Foundation representative set the stage with an overview and then handed it over to me to tell my story and make a preplanned pitch for the National Plan. Three days later, I received my first win: a sponsorship commitment from Representative Himes. A few weeks later, Senator Blumenthal committed. It was that simple. I was hooked! While I know I was just one of many people advocating for the National Plan, it felt great to be a part of it.

But then came the unfortunate news: the 117th Congress adjourned without passing the bill. We'd have to start over in 2023 with the 118th Congress. In March 2023, the bill was reintroduced and I went right back to work.

This time, the Foundation was focusing on the Senate and shared with me the senators they were targeting. Based on my earlier successes and feeling like I was a veteran of the process, I built a plan of attack. I learned that as long as I had a constituent on the call, I could set up meetings on my own with senators from any state. I focused on Connecticut, where I live, plus New York, Massachusetts, Florida, Texas and Utah—places where I had family and friends willing to join me on calls.

Of the seven senators whose offices I spoke with, three signed on, including then-Senate Majority Leader Chuck Schumer (D-NY).

*On May 23, 2024, Congress passed the
National Plan to End Parkinson's Act.*

MY VISIT TO THE CAPITOL

My work on the National Plan was just the beginning—it opened the door to new ways I could contribute. But ironically, after the bill passed, I felt an unexpected void. I'd poured myself into this effort, and now the mission was complete. I missed the momentum, the teamwork, the sense of purpose. Nothing else immediately filled that space.

And it kept not being filled until the summer of 2025, when The Michael J. Fox Foundation invited me to participate in the Parkinson's Policy Forum. A nonpartisan event, the forum is hosted by the Foundation along with the APDA, the Lewy Body Dementia Association, the Parkinson's Foundation and the Parkinson's & Movement Disorder (PMD) Alliance.

It would be the first in-person advocacy day since 2019, bringing together more than 250 patients, family members, care partners, researchers and clinicians from 45 states to call on Congress to accelerate progress toward better treatments and cures for Parkinson's.

To make the most of the opportunity, my son Zack joined me, and because he lives in Boston, we were able to attend both the Connecticut and Massachusetts meetings. A few weeks before the forum, I was asked to co-lead the Connecticut delegation and ultimately became the lead speaker in our sessions.

Over two packed days, we held five meetings with congressional staff, honored Senator Murphy (D-CT) for his leadership (see below) and connected with Parkinson's advocates from across the country—some of whom are interviewed in this book.

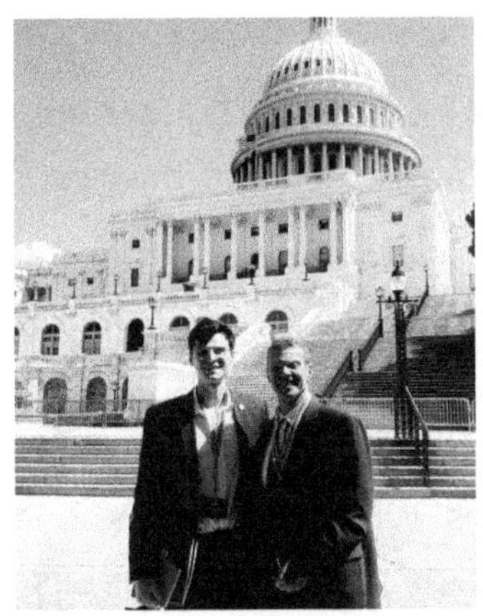 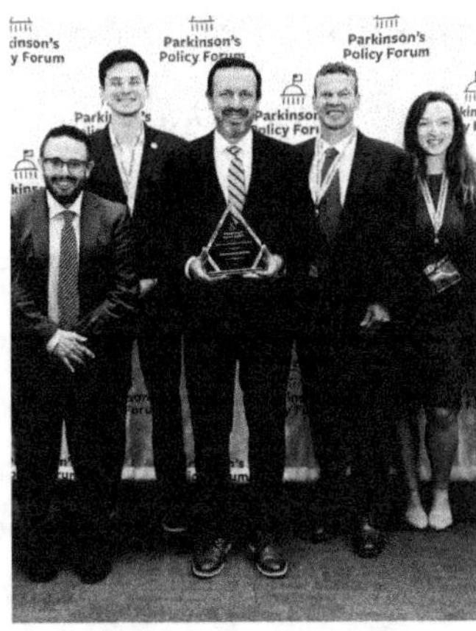

Photos from the Parkinson's Policy Forum

We were well-prepared for the meetings with talking points: seeking funding for the National Institute of Health, seating the Advisory Council for the National Parkinson's Project and supporting the effort to ban paraquat (an herbicide linked to increased risk of Parkinson's).

Depending on the session, there were up to a dozen advocates present: a mix of individuals with Parkinson's, care partners, researchers, graduate students, organization leaders, even a start-up CEO. Our messages were well-received, and we made sure there would be follow-up with members of Congress in the weeks and months ahead.

While it was a whirlwind few days, it was one of the most rewarding experiences I can remember, especially as I had Zack by my side through it all. This advocacy opportunity gave me a chance not only to make a difference but also to create lasting memories with my family. That's the heart of *Living Parkinson's*: turning challenges into opportunities to create purpose and moments that matter.

💡 EXPERT INSIGHT
The Michael J. Fox Foundation on Public Policy Advocacy

The following was adapted from content on The Michael J. Fox Foundation website and is printed with permission.

Q: What is public policy advocacy and why is it important?

MJFF: At the heart of advocacy is storytelling. Sharing your personal experience with Parkinson's brings the issue to life for lawmakers, helping them understand the urgency and human impact of policy decisions. Whether you're speaking to members of Congress or engaging with local leaders, hearing firsthand how Parkinson's impacts daily life is a powerful force for change.

Q: How does The Michael J. Fox Foundation support these advocacy efforts?

MJFF: The Foundation's Parkinson's Policy Network is our grassroots advocacy program, empowering individuals to influence public policy and accelerate progress toward a cure. Through this network, people with Parkinson's use their voices to help shape legislation and policies that directly impact the entire Parkinson's community.

Q: Who can join and how can someone get started?

MJFF: Anyone can join. No political background is needed. If you're willing to speak up, you can make a difference. As part of the Parkinson's Policy Network, you'll join a national movement working to improve care, advance research and ensure our voices are heard. You can sign up on the Foundation website.

Q: Once someone signs up, how does it work?

MJFF: Members receive policy updates and action alerts that make it easy to contact elected officials at both the federal and state levels about key Parkinson's priorities. Whether it's increasing research funding, expanding care access or raising awareness, the Policy Network gives you the tools and support to take meaningful action.

What You Can Do: Join The Michael J. Fox Foundation Policy Network

A wealth of information is available on The Michael J. Fox Foundation website (www.michaeljfox.org/advocacy). There, you'll find a list of current priorities and how to get started.

EXPLORING OTHER OPPORTUNITIES

Energized by the momentum gained from advocating for the National Plan, I began looking for other ways to contribute. Because I enjoyed telling my story, I looked for ways to engage the community with the *Living Parkinson's* message.

Over the past few years, I've spoken at events hosted by the APDA, Parkinson's Foundation and Parkinson's Body & Mind, sharing my story and encouraging others to take action. This advocacy eventually led to the seven-strategy *Living Parkinson's* program and this book.

I also began looking for other places where I could contribute and wound up enrolling in the Parkinson's Foundation's Research Advocate Program. Through the program, research advocates collaborate with scientists, industry and government leaders to make research more efficient, effective and patient-centered.

I also enrolled as a grant reviewer, evaluating and scoring annual research proposals submitted to the Parkinson's Foundation. These reviews ensure that funding goes to the studies that meet the selection criteria and have the most impact.

EXPERT INSIGHT
Evelyn Stevens and Sadie McCoy on Advocacy at the Parkinson's Foundation

Evelyn Stevens is Senior Director of Community Engagement and Sadie McCoy is the Manager of Volunteer Engagement at the Parkinson's Foundation.

Q: What types of advocacy opportunities are out there in the Parkinson's community?

EVELYN STEVENS: Advocacy looks different for everyone, just like Parkinson's disease looks different for everyone. For some, it means partnering directly with researchers and scientists to help shape clinical trials. For others, it might mean sharing their story in the community: tabling at events, attending health fairs or speaking at support groups. Some people focus on raising awareness and educating others even if they're not ready to dive into research collaboration. It all matters.

Q: What are some specific opportunities offered by the Parkinson's Foundation?

EVELYN STEVENS: The Parkinson's Foundation has both an ambassador program and a research advocate program. People often ask what the difference is. Ambassadors typically focus on broader community outreach and representing the Parkinson's Foundation at events. Research advocates, on the other hand, focus on the research process, ensuring that research reflects the real needs and priorities of people with Parkinson's.

Q: How do research advocates help advance the scientific process?

EVELYN STEVENS: Research advocates partner with scientists to design more effective research studies and clinical trials. Our program trains people with Parkinson's and their care partners on the research process so they can collaborate meaningfully with scientists. That has a real impact—it helps shape trials that deliver more value to the community. For example, advocates have helped pharmaceutical companies recognize when study visit schedules or questionnaires are too burdensome. These changes not only make trials more patient-centered, they also save time and money.

Q: What types of outreach do Parkinson's Foundation Ambassadors do?

SADIE MCCOY: Ambassadors play a key role in raising awareness at the community level. They represent the Foundation at local events like health fairs and often partner with community groups to share reliable information about Parkinson's and the resources we offer. We also provide ready-to-use slide decks on topics like "Parkinson's Basics," the "10 Early Signs of Parkinson's" and research initiatives like PD GENEration.

Q: For someone new to advocacy, where is a good place to start?

SADIE MCCOY: Volunteering at local Parkinson's Foundation events—like Moving Day or Revolutions rides—is a great first step. These roles don't require prior training and are a great way to connect with others and support the community. If someone wants to take the next step, they can enroll in our Ambassador Training Program, which prepares them to do outreach and serve as official representatives of the Foundation in their area.

What You Can Do: Become a Parkinson's Foundation Ambassador

The Parkinson's Foundation offers several meaningful ways to turn your experience into impact no matter your background, skill set or comfort level. Each program gives you the tools to impact the lives of people with Parkinson's while becoming a trusted voice in the community.

RAISING AWARENESS, FUNDING THE EFFORT

While working through established organizations and channels can be a powerful way to make your voice heard, you also can create your own grassroots projects to get the message out. The *Team Yellen* updates I periodically send to family and friends detailing our accomplishments is a platform for raising public awareness and fundraising. Every time I send out a *Team Yellen* email, I include a donation link to our personal fundraising page through either Team Fox (The Michael J. Fox Foundation) or Parkinson's Champions (Parkinson's Foundation).

These efforts have helped generate more than $5,000 annually in donations—a tribute to the family and friends in my Circle of Support (see Chapter 3). And the feedback I've received from sending the *Team Yellen* emails has been tremendously gratifying.

Everyday Advocacy

Advocacy also lives in everyday actions. Every time I share my story, I'm increasing awareness of the impact that Parkinson's has on all of us and working to create a more accurate narrative of what it means to live with the disease. I've helped newly diagnosed individuals understand what to expect, how to find care and why exercise can be a game changer. I've had conversations with friends and family about the rising prevalence of Parkinson's and the latest research into its potential environmental causes. My hope is that these small moments add up and can have an impact.

What You Can Do: Share Your Story

Educate others or fundraise at an organized event. The Parkinson's Foundation and APDA have many local events that are great opportunities to get started.

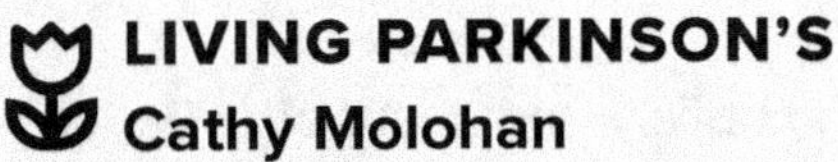 **LIVING PARKINSON'S**
Cathy Molohan

FINDING PURPOSE IN ADVOCACY

Cathy Molohan, a board member of Parkinson's Europe, is a public speaker and Parkinson's advocate based in Frankfurt, Germany.

When Cathy Molohan was diagnosed with Parkinson's at 38, it came as a shock. "I didn't have any major symptoms except for a minor tremor in my right pinky," she recalls. The doctor presented two possibilities—Parkinson's or a brain tumor—and told her to come back Monday for more tests.

For the first couple of years, Cathy focused on taking care of herself, adjusting to the news and quietly figuring out what her future might hold. "I was just trying to get used to the idea, sharing the news with friends and family," she says. At the time, she didn't see herself as an advocate. "I stayed away from the Parkinson's world because I didn't want to see what might happen to me."

It wasn't until 2016—five years after her diagnosis—that Cathy took her first step into advocacy. She attended the 4th World Parkinson Congress (WPC) in Portland in 2016, and her experience changed everything. "That was the first time I realized there was such a thing as patient advocacy," she notes.

Cathy applied to become and was accepted as an ambassador for the 5th WPC in Kyoto, Japan in 2019. Her advocacy really snowballed from there as she received inquiries from pharma companies to join their patient councils. Explains Cathy, "Drug companies are realizing they can create better solutions and trials by engaging with patients early in the process."

She also began speaking publicly—not just about Parkinson's, but about broader issues like inclusion and invisible disabilities. "My network just grew organically," Cathy says, adding that she took on new roles that amplified patient voices through conferences, advisory panels and social media. "I do some advocacy online, too. It's another way to reach people. I recently posted about the use of pesticides on golf courses and how that can cause Parkinson's."

She also completed formal training to become a Parkinson's advocate, which gave her the tools to speak confidently in policy settings and on advisory panels. It helped her understand how to represent the community effectively and share more than just her own story.

Her work has grown to encompass a larger scale. "I work with an organization in Europe called the European Federation of Neurological Associations," she adds. "They really try to push policymakers in Brussels to a new level to get neurological diseases more firmly on the EU agenda."

For Cathy, advocacy became a pathway toward connection and purpose. To someone newly diagnosed or anyone curious about getting involved, she offers this advice: "Find something that resonates with you and aligns with your strengths. Are you a good public speaker? Maybe you're great with technology and could help design solutions with med-tech companies. Or maybe you simply want to connect. Start by showing up in the community.

"What drives me is purpose—the feeling that I'm part of something bigger and I'm doing something that matters. It empowers me to do something I love."

SOCIAL MEDIA AS A VEHICLE FOR ADVOCACY

You can't discuss advocacy today without including the role of social media—it's become one of the most powerful tools we have to raise awareness. Both Instagram and Facebook are popular platforms for sharing experiences, challenges and solutions to common problems.

There are Parkinson's advocates with tens of thousands of followers on Instagram who are posting regularly on what living with the disease really looks like. A quick search for "Parkinson's" in Facebook groups returns more than 50 communities—some with more than 10,000 members—focused on every possible aspect of the disease. If you *don't* see your interest represented, you can create a group!

These platforms amplify your voice, giving it reach. Whether you're sharing your daily workout, posting a fundraiser link, offering advice on a specific topic or simply commenting on someone else's post, you're advocating. You're shaping the narrative. And that matters.

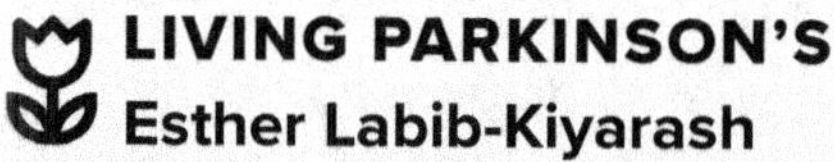

LIVING PARKINSON'S
Esther Labib-Kiyarash

FROM FINDING HER VOICE TO BECOMING ONE

Esther Labib-Kiyarash, a healthcare administrator and mother turned TikTok influencer and advocate, is based in El Paso, Texas.

Esther Labib-Kiyarash's path to diagnosis was anything but simple—what began as persistent pain and strange sensations turned into a frustrating cycle of misdiagnosis, second opinions and emotional whiplash. It wasn't until she reached the Mayo Clinic and was seen by a movement disorder specialist that her Parkinson's diagnosis was confirmed.

What came next surprised even her.

Esther didn't wait long to speak up—within a week of her diagnosis, she picked up her phone and started recording TikTok videos. "I probably made my first Parkinson's video by the end of that week," she notes, adding that for her, the choice wasn't about building a following, it was about survival. "I felt really alone. I didn't have anybody to talk to about this except other people online."

At first, Esther imagined a kind of visual journal—an honest, unfiltered chronicle of her life from diagnosis onward. "I had this idea that I was going to document my decline—

like a digital photo book or a baby book, but for Parkinson's."

Her goal was raw visibility, to show what Parkinson's looked like from the beginning, not just in the later stages. "I wanted it to be what I had been looking for."

Over time, Esther realized that her videos were doing more than just giving her a voice—they were giving others a mirror. People began messaging her to say, "That's me! I've felt that, too."

In documenting her own experience, Esther was helping others understand *theirs*. She unknowingly had filled a void for connection among those living with Parkinson's who were searching for someone like them. Her diagnosis video alone reached a quarter of a million views.

But the impact didn't stop there. Esther saw that her content also helped people without Parkinson's—those who had never seen it up close. "Before, someone might've seen a person trip or fall off a curb and assumed they were drunk. Now, they might think, 'Maybe that's Parkinson's.'"

Through simple, honest clips, she was shifting public perception, building empathy and expanding awareness. She later added Facebook and Instagram accounts to reach other demographics.

For those considering social media advocacy, Esther has practical advice: "You don't have to start by posting. Just reply to people. Join the conversation. That's how it starts. Over time, you might feel ready to share your own story."

She reminds people not to overlook local connections, either. "Social media is powerful, but sometimes the most meaningful impact comes from showing up in your own community."

Esther didn't set out to become a champion for others—she just put herself out there, unfiltered, and now helps others recognize their own voice.

You can find Esther on TikTok at @estherlabibkiyara and on Instagram at @shakinginmyboots1, where she continues to share life with Parkinson's one moment at a time.

WAYS TO TAKE ACTION

Advocacy is one of the most rewarding ways to make a difference. It enables you to use your voice, experience and passion to support others, influence change and help raise money for research. It's incredibly satisfying—knowing that you've "moved the ball forward" brings a sense of accomplishment and purpose that's hard to match.

There's no one-size-fits-all approach. You can choose the forms of advocacy that align with your strengths, interests and opportunities. Here are some impactful ways to get started:

- ▸ **USE YOUR VOICE:** Share your story in writing, or in a support group or online to educate others, reduce stigma and inspire connection.

- ▸ **SUPPORT OTHERS:** Be a peer guide, mentor someone who's newly diagnosed or help friends and family better understand Parkinson's.

- ▸ **GET INVOLVED LOCALLY:** Attend or volunteer at local events or serve as a Parkinson's Foundation ambassador.

- ▸ **INFLUENCE RESEARCH:** Become a research advocate or grant reviewer to help shape the science that shapes our care.

▶ **PUSH FOR POLICY:** Contact lawmakers, support legislation and join national efforts like The Michael J. Fox Foundation's Parkinson's Policy Network to drive systemic change.

What You Can Do: Pick One Advocacy Option and Get Started

It doesn't need to be a major commitment—You can participate in a local event and do some fundraising, or maybe just spend some time researching what's available to you. Small steps...

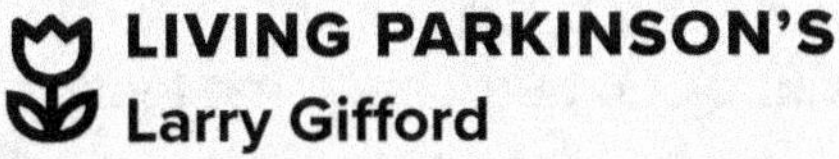 **LIVING PARKINSON'S**
Larry Gifford

SPEAKING UP, SPARKING CHANGE

Larry Gifford, president and co-founder of PD Avengers, is a radio professional and host of multiple podcasts who's based in Vancouver, Canada.

When Larry Gifford was diagnosed with Parkinson's at age 45, he wasn't just stunned, he was frustrated—not just at the diagnosis, but at the world around him. "There was no urgency," he recalls. "No one seemed to be in a hurry to do anything about this disease."

That frustration quickly turned into action. Larry didn't have a roadmap, but he had a voice and he started using it. He began telling his story through a podcast, and what started as an effort to process his own experience became something much bigger.

"I realized I wasn't the only one feeling this way. There were people all over the world who were also living with Parkinson's—and also ready to do something."

Those conversations planted the seeds of what would become the PD Avengers, a global alliance of people with Parkinson's, care partners and allies working together to end the disease. Larry co-founded the organization in 2020, officially launching in 2021 with a bold mission: spark action, raise awareness, eliminate preventable causes, expand access to care and accelerate a cure. "One voice can make noise," he says. "But thousands of voices? That's when things start to change."

Larry's story isn't about strategy or structure, it's about energy. Advocacy for him wasn't a calculated career move—it was something he had to do. "I just couldn't sit back and wait. So I started speaking out. That was the beginning."

For Larry, the power of advocacy is deeply personal: "It gives you back a sense of control. Of purpose." That feeling of empowerment has been one of the most transformative parts of his journey. "When you're living with a progressive disease, there's so much you can't change. But when you speak up—when you act—you remember you still have a say."

His advocacy hasn't just changed how he lives, it has connected him to people around the world who also refuse to sit quietly. Through campaigns like Spark the Night—when more than 500 top landmarks around the world were lit up in blue on World Parkinson's Day—the PD Avengers are building a global network: raising awareness, fighting stigma and showing the world that people with Parkinson's are not invisible.

One thing that gives him hope is seeing patient advocates now being invited into research discussions and grant reviews, places where their voices were once absent. "That's what change looks like," he says. "Not just being seen, but being included."

For those who have been newly diagnosed, Larry doesn't hand out advice, he shares experience: "Just start where you are. Maybe it's telling one person. Maybe it's asking a question your doctor doesn't expect. Maybe it's just saying, 'This matters to me.' That's advocacy, too."

Being an advocate is more than just action, it's an identity, Larry observes. "With a disease that can so often make people feel powerless, advocacy becomes a way to take some of that power back."

His story is a reminder that advocacy doesn't have to be loud or polished or public, it just has to be honest. It's about showing up, for yourself and for others, in whatever way you can. "One person's voice can be the spark for real change."

THE HIDDEN POWER OF ADVOCACY

Advocacy isn't *one* thing—it's anything that uses your experience and voice to make a difference.

Personal Benefits of Being an Advocate

BENEFIT	WHY IT MATTERS
Renewed Sense of Purpose	Advocacy gives people a mission, something larger to work on. A sense of meaning can be especially valuable after diagnosis.
Increased Self-Efficacy	Action builds confidence in your ability to influence outcomes. Small wins reinforce your capacity to lead and problem-solve.
Stronger Social Connections	Advocacy opens doors to new friendships and community. Working with others at local events fosters camaraderie.

BENEFIT	WHY IT MATTERS
Cognitive Engagement	Participating in meetings challenges your mind in positive ways. Activity supports brain health and keeps you mentally active.
Satisfaction of Helping Others	Few things are as gratifying as knowing you helped someone. You may help someone who's newly diagnosed adjust faster.

Conclusion

Advocacy has become more than just something I do—it's become part of how I live with Parkinson's. It's helped me stay connected, engaged and focused on what I can do. In short, it's a big part of fueling my self-efficacy. Whether we're talking to a government official, posting on social media or just offering support to someone who's newly diagnosed, we're making a difference. I've seen firsthand how one voice shared at the right time can move things forward.

Looking Ahead: Strategy #7 – Research

Advocacy is one way to create change; participating in research is another. In the next chapter, we'll explore how people with Parkinson's can play a direct role in driving scientific discovery. You'll learn how research participation can lead to not just a future of better treatments and progress toward a cure for Parkinson's, but how it can benefit your own journey as well.

TAKEAWAYS/ACTION PLAN

CHAPTER 7

RESEARCH

Help Advance the Science

Each person who joins a study
helps move science forward.

WHAT YOU'LL LEARN IN THIS CHAPTER

- ▶ Why participating in research matters—and how it can directly benefit you
- ▶ The difference between observational and interventional studies
- ▶ How to find a study that fits your comfort level
- ▶ The personal impact of contributing to science
- ▶ Tools and resources to help you get started

One of the first thoughts anyone who's heard the words "You have Parkinson's" has is, "We need a cure." While finding one won't be easy, it can't even *begin* without research. And research depends on people willing to step up and participate.

At any given time, hundreds of studies are actively underway—not just to find a cure, but to discover earlier detection tools, better treatments and new ways to improve quality of life. When you take part in a clinical trial, a data study or even a patient survey, you're doing more than just helping science, you're taking an active role in shaping the future.

Beyond your contribution to science, participation can be deeply personal. It can offer purpose, connection and sometimes even early access to tools or insights that could help you live better today, not just in the future.

One of the major advocacy goals discussed in the previous chapter was raising awareness, because awareness drives funding, funding fuels research and research will ultimately lead to winning the battle against Parkinson's.

This chapter will help you understand what types of research opportunities are available, where to find them and what to consider when determining which ones are the right ones for you. *Living Parkinson's* means not just navigating what *is* but also helping to build what *could be*.

MY INTRODUCTION TO RESEARCH

I didn't set out to become a research participant. But like much about living with Parkinson's, an opportunity arose to become part of something bigger, and it unexpectedly changed the course of my journey from the moment I said yes.

In November 2020, more than a year after my diagnosis, I received an email inviting me to join the Fox Insight study. This online study collects self-reported data about health experiences from those with and without Parkinson's every 90 days. I decided to join. It just involved completing an online survey and would accelerate research, so why not?

Within days of filling out that survey, I received a second email inviting me to the Fox Insight Genetic Substudy, launched in partnership with personal genetics company 23andMe. This study would link genetic data from a DNA collection kit with the information I had already provided to further benefit research. I had considered genetic testing in the past, so I opted in. (Remember my passion for collecting and analyzing data? Not to mention I'd get a free genetics report out of it.)

I had come to appreciate not just the value of contributing but also the insights I was gaining about my condition.

In February 2021, I received my 23andMe Parkinson's Disease Report, which in bold letters said, "Steven, you do not have the two genetic variants we tested. Zero variants detected in the LRRK2 and GBA genes." The report struck a chord with the problem-solver and science geek in me.

I also downloaded a more general 23andMe report with even more genetic information. I think this really opened my eyes to the type of information I could receive and how much better equipped I could be in my Parkinson's battle.

Also that February, I received an email inviting me to join the Fox Parkinson's Progression Markers Initiative (PPMI), another long-term observational study. This time I joined right away.

In March 2021, a researcher on the PPMI team referred me to the PD GENEration study, another global research study offering free genetic testing for people with Parkinson's. I learned more on the Parkinson's Foundation website and decided to enroll. This would go beyond the two genes I had previously been tested for and would check for five more that were associated with the disease (PD GENEration results have found that approximately 12-13% of people with Parkinson's carry a genetic variant in one of the seven primary Parkinson's-related genes[20]). A few months later, I received my results and found out that I didn't have any of the genes associated with Parkinson's.

By 2022, I had come to appreciate not just the value of contributing but also the insights I was gaining about my condition. What additional opportunities were out there? That's when I began looking for more studies and found CenterWatch, a website that lists clinical trials.

I learned that research studies generally fall into two broad categories: observational, where researchers gather data without introducing any changes, and interventional, which tests the efficacy of a specific drug or treatment (see next page). As a participant, your role is meaningful in both. While you might choose one or the other based on your comfort level, health status or personal goals, both contribute to progress.

What You Can Do: Enroll in the Parkinson's Progression Markers Initiative (PPMI)

The PPMI is a landmark study by The Michael J. Fox Foundation. It gathers information over time to learn more about how brain disease starts and changes, and how to stop it. You can start by sharing information online, and if you're interested, you can provide biological samples. You can find out how to enroll on the Foundation's website.

TYPES OF RESEARCH STUDIES

Observational Studies

In an observational study, researchers track participants over time to see how certain factors—like lifestyle, symptoms or biomarkers—relate to outcomes.

> **EXAMPLE:** A study that follows people with Parkinson's for five years to track how their sleep patterns relate to disease progression.

> **GOAL:** Identify patterns, correlations or risk factors.

Think of it like being a "research witness"—you're not asked to change anything, just to share what's already happening in your body or life. Observational studies help researchers understand the natural course of Parkinson's and often inform the design of future interventional trials.

Interventional Study

In an interventional study, researchers actively introduce a treatment, behavior or therapy to see if it makes a difference.

> **EXAMPLE:** A clinical trial that tests whether a new drug slows motor decline, with participants assigned to different groups (e.g., drug vs. placebo).

> **GOAL:** Test cause and effect—does the intervention help?

Here, you're not just observed, you're part of testing something new that might help you or others. Interventional studies take the next step: evaluating whether an idea or approach can actually improve quality of life or slow disease progression.

MY FIRST INTERVENTIONAL STUDY

As I searched for new studies to participate in, one caught my eye because of its focus on exercise: Pre-Active PD, run out of Teachers College at Columbia University. The study investigated the effects of occupational therapist-guided coaching on improving self-efficacy, motivation and physical activity in people with Parkinson's. In May 2022, I enrolled and worked one-on-one virtually with an occupational therapist. It was like a master class in exercise for Parkinson's.

In August 2022, my movement disorder specialist at Yale told me about another opportunity: a study led by Dr. Sule Tinaz exploring how mental imagery training could affect motor function and brain plasticity. I joined the following January because I saw an opportunity to learn skills that could improve my motor function.

The study involved multiple one-hour sessions in an MRI scanner, where I practiced mental simulations of movement (thankfully, I'm not claustrophobic). Ironically, most of my conversations with Dr. Tinaz were about her other exercise-related studies—proof that Parkinson's research, like the disease itself, doesn't always follow a straight line.

What started with one click has turned into an ongoing commitment.

Soon after, I joined Engage-PD, another Teachers College study evaluating the benefits of physical activity coaching. This time I worked with a physical therapist, and again I learned new ways to use exercise to manage my Parkinson's. As I built relationships with the Teachers College team, they began reaching out with more opportunities. In October 2023, I joined a biomechanics study, where I wore sensors to analyze my movements: walking, standing, getting up from the floor and more.

In 2024, a different type of study caught my attention, especially given the growing research around the gut-brain connection. The Parkinson's Disease Biomarkers in Nerve Cells in the Gut study involved an analysis of my microbiome and the collection of tissue samples during a routine colonoscopy. Since I was due for the procedure anyway, I saw it as an opportunity to contribute while learning more about my own microbiome.

I also participated in a few other studies along the way. In June 2024, I joined a Boston University study on speech and motor outcomes. And in March 2025, I enrolled in the Yale-Harvard Biomarker Study—a long-term project that collects biological samples in seven visits over 20 years for a research tissue bank in support of future studies. These studies don't provide me with any personal data, but they give me the satisfaction of knowing I'm part of the broader fight.

What started with one click has turned into an ongoing commitment.

EXPERT INSIGHT
Roy Alcalay on Research Participation

Dr. Roy Alcalay, MD, MS, is chief of the Movement Disorders Division at Tel Aviv Sourasky Medical Center and also affiliated with Columbia University, where he holds a part-time associate professorship. His work centers on genetic and biological subtypes of Parkinson's with an emphasis on early biomarkers, patient-centered studies and clinical trials design.

Q: Why should those with Parkinson's consider participating in research?

DR. ALCALAY: It's personal, but many do it to help move science forward. When you have Parkinson's, you're in a race and you want science to win. Participating in research—whether by sharing your data, giving blood samples or taking part in clinical assessments—helps improve the odds that science can win.

Q: What are the personal benefits of participating in observational studies?

DR. ALCALAY: Empowerment is a big one. You have control over what you join and how involved you are. It's an active way to fight back. You're not just living with Parkinson's, you're helping to shape its future. Another important factor is a new trend called "return of results," where participants can receive their personal data, such as genetic information or biomarker results, from the studies they take part in. This shift is driven by the belief that sharing results empowers participants, encourages involvement and fosters proactive health decisions.

Q: Why might someone consider an interventional study?

DR. ALCALAY: Clinical trials may give participants early access to new therapies—sometimes years before FDA approval—along with careful monitoring. Even when there's no guarantee of benefit and you could be in the placebo group, you get an added level of care by being in the study. And being part of something bigger, something that could help others, is meaningful.

Q: Where would someone look to learn about current studies?

DR. ALCALAY: You can start by asking your local treatment center—they often run or can refer you to active studies in your area. There are also an increasing number of online studies, which you can find using a search engine like The Michael J. Fox Foundation's Fox Trial Finder, matching participants to trials based on location and eligibility. It's a great starting point if you're unsure where to begin.

Q: What would you say to someone who's considering participation?

DR. ALCALAY: Research is always voluntary. You're not a test subject, you're a partner. Every contribution—no matter how small—helps move the needle. You can always say no, but you also might find real purpose in saying yes.

CHOOSING THE RIGHT STUDIES

As I explored the wide range of studies out there, I began to see just how many opportunities exist, each with different criteria for joining and each requiring different levels of involvement. Now whenever I come across an interesting study, I evaluate it based on my current condition.

So far, I haven't enrolled in interventional studies that involve drug trials. I don't feel that my Parkinson's is at a point where pursuing an alternative treatment to my current medications and exercise is necessary. That said, as my Parkinson's situation changes, so may my decisions.

The choices I make are what I believe are right for me at the time based on my current condition. For example, I recently found a study involving multiple PET scans using a radioactive tracer. The disclosure form stated, "The amount of additional radiation you will receive from participating in this study is equal to about 12 years' worth of natural background radiation." That concerned me....

I talked it through with my movement disorder specialist and a few friends who are physicians. One doctor friend explained, "These tracers are primarily used for detecting cancer. In that case, the concern with the radiation exposure is secondary to the cancer diagnosis." As much as I wanted to participate, it didn't feel right for me. Passing on studies like this one is a very difficult and individual decision.

The takeaway? Like much of a Parkinson's journey, everyone's path is unique and these decisions are personal. It's important to weigh the risks and rewards in your own mind, talk with your care team and make choices that align with your comfort level and priorities. Research participation can be incredibly rewarding—but it should never come at the expense of your peace of mind.

What You Can Do: Plan Ahead – What Is Your Comfort Zone?

If you're considering research participation, it helps to know your limits ahead of time. What are you willing to do? Where would you draw the line? Thinking through those boundaries can help you make quicker, more confident decisions to find the research study that's right for you.

SEARCH TOOLS AND VIRTUAL OPTIONS

I've also discovered a few great resources for finding studies; I touched on a few already. ClinicalTrials.gov and The Michael J. Fox Foundation's Trial Finder are both user-friendly platforms that list a wide range of opportunities. While using these online tools, I learned about virtual studies (research you can participate in from home). That's how I found online studies like PD GENEration, PPMI Online and Fox Insight.

I also came across additional virtual research projects through institutions like the University of Delaware, Stanford University, Tel Aviv University, University of Rochester, George Washington University and McGill University. Each offers another way to get involved and stay connected to the front lines of Parkinson's research—no travel required.

🌷 LIVING PARKINSON'S
Kevin Kwok

TURNING DIAGNOSIS INTO PURPOSE THROUGH RESEARCH

Kevin Kwok, a retired biopharmaceutical operations and consulting executive, is a Parkinson's patient advocate based in Boulder, Colorado.

Kevin Kwok was at the height of his career when Parkinson's disease entered his life. At age 48, while on a business trip to Singapore, he experienced extreme rigidity in his neck and shoulders and feared he'd had a stroke. He returned home, where his primary care physician immediately suspected Parkinson's and confirmed the diagnosis with a neurologist.

Instead of retreating, Kevin leaned in. With a background in pharmaceutical research and patient engagement, he decided early on to become part of the solution. Inspired by how patient communities in cancer and HIV had influenced research and care, Kevin asked his neurologist to help him get involved with Parkinson's research. She responded, "What do you mean?" and he said, "I'm not sure, but I just know I want to play a role."

Kevin's research journey has been wide-ranging. He's participated in everything from simple genetic studies and symptom tracking surveys to high-intensity interventional trials. On the observational side, he's contributed to studies like the Parkinson's Progression Markers Initiative (PPMI). He's also taken part in genetic research and meditation trials. These forms of research are vital—helping scientists identify patterns, understand progression and improve study design.

Kevin also has taken part in interventional studies, including a five-year collaboration on adaptive deep brain stimulation (DBS). This groundbreaking technology adjusts to patient needs in real time, an advance Kevin helped shape with his feedback and data. "Fifteen years after I started, that version of DBS got approved. To know I had a hand in that is incredibly rewarding."

He also joined a study based on regenerative blood therapy concepts that infused plasma from younger donors into older Parkinson's patients. Another trial, TOPAZ, investigated fracture prevention and brought treatment to his home, showing how research can literally meet people where they live.

Kevin now serves on the Steering Committee for the LoCaMOTE trial, which explores a hypothesis drawn from epidemiology: While no one would ever recommend smoking, smokers appear less likely to develop Parkinson's. LoCaMOTE will test hypoxia (low-oxygen states) as a potential protective mechanism. As Kevin puts it, "LoCaMOTE is a novel shot at changing the playing field by building on what's been observed."

The benefits Kevin has received are substantial. First, there's the personal empowerment. "In a world where you're dealing with a disease that feels like it's out of your control, being involved in research may be the highest form of control we have," he says. It gives Kevin a sense of purpose and direction, and he's also benefited from exposure to cutting-edge treatments and a deeper knowledge of his condition.

Research has kept him intellectually engaged and emotionally grounded. "I stay mentally active because I'm constantly thinking about what's next," he observes, adding that even when results aren't immediate, the process is rewarding. "You rarely do a study and get an answer right away, but every study adds a piece to the puzzle."

He encourages others to start small. "You don't have to do everything. Share a saliva sample. Try a virtual study. Doing something helps the science—and it helps you. And find yourself a trusted guide, learn what's available and don't get paralyzed by information overload. Being informed might be the most powerful thing you can do, even if you decide not to participate."

THE UNEXPECTED PERSONAL REWARDS OF PARTICIPATION

While participating in research gives me real satisfaction in knowing I'm contributing—playing even a small part in the bigger picture—I've found a few unexpected personal benefits along the way. Two that particularly stand out are:

- ▶ Gaining baseline health data that may help me in the future
- ▶ Educating myself more and building relationships with researchers

The Power of Baseline Data

One of the most tangible personal benefits of participating in multiple studies is the ability to gather detailed baseline data on myself—something I believe is incredibly valuable.

Through these studies, I now have multiple fMRIs of my brain, extensive results from cognitive testing, biomechanical movement analyses and even a full microbiome profile. I've essentially built a personal health database that goes far deeper than what I'd get in a typical clinical visit.

It's already helped. In 2024, I began experiencing some minor pain in my side and noticed my posture shifting—one shoulder was higher than the other. It concerned me. So I reached back out to the Teachers College biomechanics lab, where I'd participated in the study the year before. I wanted to see if they could reevaluate me and see if anything had changed in my biomechanics. They were happy to invite me in to re-run the previous analysis they had done a year earlier.

We compared the results to my original data from 2023. Fortunately, there hadn't been any meaningful change—but the real value was in having the baseline for comparison. Without that original dataset, I'd be guessing.

And who knows? If future research confirms a stronger link between gut health and Parkinson's, the microbiome profile I received in 2024 might become even more useful, for me as well as for others.

Anytime I get screened for a research study where I see an opportunity to capture baseline data, I make sure to ask the study coordinator if it's available to me. In at least one case, it wasn't part of the standard procedure, but they agreed to provide me with my raw data.

What You Can Do: Learn About Your Condition

Think about the information you'd like to have about yourself. Then use your desired data as a guide to look for a study that might provide you with that information.

Gaining Insights and Building Relationships

Another unexpected benefit of research participation has been the relationships I've built with researchers along the way. Whenever I participate in a study, I try to understand the deeper purpose behind it: What are they trying to learn and why does this question matter for Parkinson's? That curiosity has turned every study into a learning opportunity.

But it's not just what I've learned, it's who I've met. I've developed connections with some of the researchers running these programs, relationships that may prove valuable in the future. Whether I have a follow-up question, want to revisit a lab for updated data or simply need guidance, I now have people I can reach out to—people I trust.

In fact, when I experienced the minor side pain in 2024, in addition to getting reevaluated at the biomechanics lab at Teacher's College, I reached out to the physical therapist I had worked with in the Engage-PD study. A Parkinson's specialist, she invited me up to her lab at Marist College for an evaluation and wound up prescribing certain exercises.

In Chapter 5, I highlighted the importance of building a network. Researchers can be part of that network, too. They're not just running studies, they're partners in the pursuit of answers. And for those of us living with Parkinson's, that's a partnership worth cultivating!

What You Can Do: Identify Your Areas of Interest

Are there specific areas within the Parkinson's research realm that interest you (e.g., genetics, gut-brain connection)? Look for a study that focuses on that aspect of Parkinson's and use it as an opportunity to meet researchers and learn from them.

💡 EXPERT INSIGHT
Lori Quinn on Exercise-Based Studies

Dr. Lori Quinn, EdD, PT, is Director of the Neurorehabil-itation Research Lab at Teachers College at Columbia University. Her research centers on helping people with neurological conditions—including Parkinson's—sustain long-term engagement in physical activity.

Q: What kinds of Parkinson's studies have you led?

DR. QUINN: We design and test physical activity interventions that support people in staying active over time. That includes coaching programs delivered by occupational or physical therapists rooted in behavior change theory. Our studies are less about testing a new exercise itself and more about helping people follow through with what works. It's about giving people the tools to build habits that last.

Q: How do you decide what to study?

DR. QUINN: I look at where the need is. There's a lot of evidence that exercise helps, but a big limitation is that people with Parkinson's often don't stay engaged. They might start strong but then drop off. That's true for all of us in some ways. So I focus on what helps people stick with exercise long-term and how we can make that support more accessible.

Q: Why do most people join your studies?

DR. QUINN: Most want to give back, to be part of something bigger. But many are also looking for help, for tools and strategies that make exercise more manageable. I want participants to walk away with something tangible they can use in daily life. That might be a new way to track their activity or a personalized strategy to stay motivated. It's research, but it's also about building skills.

Q: What have you seen people gain from participating?

DR. QUINN: Confidence. Knowledge. A greater sense of control. When people find an approach that works for them, they feel more capable—not just physically, but mentally and emotionally, too. That's powerful. I've seen people take what they learned and apply it long after the study ends.

Q: What would you say to someone considering a study?

DR. QUINN: Every study is different, and not all of them are right for everyone. But ask questions! If it feels like a good fit, it can be incredibly rewarding. Participating doesn't mean giving up control—it often *builds* it. You're helping science move forward, yes, but you're also helping yourself.

SMARTPHONE APPS: RESEARCH IN YOUR POCKET

You don't always need to visit a lab or hospital to contribute to research. Increasingly, smartphone apps and online platforms are being used to collect valuable data from people with Parkinson's. These digital studies are almost always observational and offer easy ways to get involved, often through simple daily tasks, symptom tracking or cognitive games.

For example, the StrivePD® Apple Watch and mobile app passively collect tremor and dyskinesia data, delivering insights into mobility and motor symptoms.

These apps not only support researchers, but also give you new ways to understand your own patterns, helping to track symptoms, exercise, sleep and more. Digital studies make research accessible to more people, especially those who don't live near a research center or who prefer to contribute on their own schedule.

Conclusion

Research, for me, has become more than just a way to contribute—it's a way to continue learning and meeting more people with a common goal: beating Parkinson's.

Whether I'm filling out an online survey, giving a blood sample or wearing a device that tracks my movement, I know I'm doing something that matters and may provide tangible benefits in the future. In a Parkinson's journey where so much can feel out of your control, that kind of purpose goes a long way.

Looking Ahead: Living the Journey with Positivity

We've now explored the full arc of *Living Parkinson's*, from attitude and education to support, exercise, wellness, advocacy and research. Each chapter has offered tools to help you shape your own path forward.

But this journey isn't just about strategies—it's about taking control, redefining your purpose and winning your battle. In the final section, we'll look to the future: how to move forward with a sense of positivity that isn't forced, which is the true spirit of *Living Parkinson's*.

TAKEAWAYS/ACTION PLAN

Live the Journey with Positivity

You didn't get to choose the
diagnosis, but you get to choose
how you respond.

Writing this book has been one of the hardest things I've ever done—and one of the most rewarding. I'm a private person who usually keeps personal battles to myself. But telling my story in the hope of helping others has pushed me, challenged me and, yes, fueled my self-efficacy. The chance to meet inspiring Parkinson's warriors has reminded me why this fight matters.

Through it all, I've continued to learn. The experts I interviewed reinforced a powerful message: *Parkinson's is manageable.* The global organizations I spoke with are working hard not only to support people today, but to drive progress toward better treatments and scientific advances.

And some of my biggest takeaways came from the people with Parkinson's I met along the way who, despite the challenges, consistently expressed resilience, determination and hope. Their stories didn't just inform this book, they helped shape it.

And more than anything, the people I interviewed confirmed my resolve that the *Living Parkinson's* formula can work. The seven strategies aren't theory, they're tools that real people are already using to live fuller, stronger, more purposeful lives—myself included.

THE ROLE OF GRATITUDE

As I met more people *Living Parkinson's*, I came upon a surprising paradox: The most powerful emotion I consistently heard from others on this journey was gratitude for what they have and for what they can control. Gratitude doesn't erase the challenges of Parkinson's, but it can reframe them. It's not about pretending everything's easy, it's about recognizing what's still good.

> The most powerful emotion I consistently heard from others on this journey was gratitude for what they have and for what they can control.

I want to acknowledge that expressing gratitude isn't equally easy for everyone. Each of our journeys with Parkinson's is unique. For some, the road is more difficult and the good moments are harder to find. But wherever you *can* find gratitude, it can be a source of strength.

The more I've embraced the strategies I've described in this book—shifting my mindset, learning what matters, building my team, fighting back with exercise, caring for my body, striving for progress and participating in research—the more I've realized how much there still is to be thankful for. Gratitude, in that sense, is both a mindset and a reward. It doesn't arrive passively, it grows through action.

CALMING UNCERTAINTY WITH PURPOSE

Living with Parkinson's means living with uncertainty. There's no fixed timeline, no clear map, no guaranteed outcome for any of us—and each of our paths will be different. But uncertainty doesn't have to mean fear. In fact, it can be a catalyst, a moment in life to focus on what we *can* control: our mindset, our choices and how we respond to challenges. While we may not control the course of the disease, we *do* control how we respond to it.

That's where purpose comes in. Purpose gives direction to our efforts. But having purpose is personal and is about doing what gives you meaning. Ironically, getting Parkinson's gave me a new purpose: beating it. And writing this book has given me purpose, with the ultimate goal of making a difference. I want to provide a path for others with Parkinson's to fight back, take control and live a fulfilling life.

PARTING THOUGHTS

This book isn't a roadmap to perfection, it's an invitation to live the best life you can while still reaching for more. For those of us with Parkinson's, we are in a long-term battle for our lives. But that battle can be fought with clarity, courage and purpose.

I opened Chapter 1 by challenging a sentiment I've heard many times: "Don't let Parkinson's define you." I want to close on that same thought, because for me, Parkinson's isn't something I can ignore or set aside. It's with me 24/7/365. Parkinson's and I are inseparable until the day I can declare victory.

Until then, I will never stop fighting. And I hope you won't, either.

#NEVERGIVEUP   #BEATPD   #LIVINGPARKINSONS

Living Parkinson's Around the World

According to the Parkinson's Foundation, only about 10% of the 10 million people living with Parkinson's worldwide are in the United States. That statistic reminds me that while my experiences (and much of this book) are shaped by the U.S. healthcare system and cultural landscape, Parkinson's is global.

With that in mind, I reached out to a handful of leading researchers, advocates and organizations in other parts of the world to better understand the larger landscape. These one-on-one conversations certainly don't represent every perspective, but they offer some valuable insights on unique regional challenges as well as the common goals and values we all share.

By sharing these global perspectives, my hope is that readers around the world can see what opportunities exist in their own regions, whether that's to get involved, to advocate, to participate in research or simply to be part of the larger Parkinson's movement. Understanding how others are approaching the same challenges helps us learn from one another and reminds us that every contribution, no matter where it comes from, moves the cause forward.

Africa

Dr. Natasha Fothergill-Misbah, Transforming Parkinson's Care in Africa (TraPCAf) Research Associate, Newcastle University

Omotola Thomas, founder of Parkinson's Africa

Talk about the mission of Parkinson's Africa.

Parkinson's Africa was founded on the simple premise that no one should have to face Parkinson's alone. Our mission is to transform the Parkinson's disease landscape across the 54 countries that make up the African continent, community by community, into societies where those affected have access to quality healthcare, research, support, information and educational resources. We aim to bring about a paradigm shift in the way Parkinson's is perceived across Africa, to reduce the burden of stigma associated with the disease and to empower the African Parkinson's community.

Together—with compassion, determination and collaboration—we believe we can dismantle the stigma, close the information gap and empower every African impacted by Parkinson's to live well despite the challenges the condition may bring.

What are some of the key challenges for the Parkinson's community in Africa?

Awareness, diagnosis and access to treatment are the most urgent challenges. In many regions across Africa, Parkinson's disease is virtually unknown, not only among the public but also among healthcare providers and policymakers. This lack of awareness contributes to widespread stigma—it's sometimes linked to supernatural beliefs—and results in people going undiagnosed for years. Even if diagnosed, medication is often unavailable or unaffordable, and the general health literacy around managing Parkinson's is very low. As a result, many people suffer untreated for years, unaware they even have the disease.

Tell us a little more about the issues specific to Africa.

Parkinson's frequently goes undiagnosed—often for eight to ten years *after* symptoms appear—because of a shortage of specialists and limited knowledge among frontline health workers. Many African countries have only a handful of neurologists, if any. Even when diagnosed, people often lack access to medication or the knowledge of non-drug interventions. It's estimated that 60% to 70% of people living with Parkinson's in Africa don't know they have it. In many communities, people living with symptoms are stigmatized or forced into isolation due to misconceptions about the disease.

How can people with Parkinson's contribute to the effort?

Despite having limited resources, people with Parkinson's can and do contribute. Advocacy is emerging through awareness campaigns, support groups and storytelling. As part of the TraPCAf project, we have developed documentary films in countries like Kenya and Tanzania that can be shared locally and globally to reduce stigma and increase understanding. Support groups are especially powerful—they fill critical gaps left by under-resourced health systems and offer spaces for education, community and advocacy. Efforts are also underway to pair support groups with donor partners to improve access to medication.

Australia

Emma Collin, Chief Executive Officer, Fight Parkinson's

Tell us about Fight Parkinson's and its mission.

Fight Parkinson's, based in Victoria, is a leading Australian organization dedicated to improving the lives of people living with Parkinson's and related conditions. Our mission is to enable people to live well today through evidence-based health services, education and peer support—all while driving advocacy, research and innovation toward prevention and ultimately freedom from Parkinson's. We provide free, expert information and tailored advice through our multidisciplinary health team, and we connect thousands of people across the state and beyond through our peer-support networks. Our online programs ensure that even those outside Victoria can benefit from quality education and connection.

What are the main challenges facing people with Parkinson's in Australia?

Awareness and access to care remain two big challenges. Around 200,000 Australians, including 50,000 Victorians, live with Parkinson's, but diagnosis can be delayed and care is inconsistent, especially outside major cities. People in rural and regional areas often struggle to see movement disorder specialists or access Parkinson's-informed therapies such as physiotherapy, speech therapy or occupational therapy. Geography, income and policy settings also affect access to care, with many unable to afford private therapy or travel long distances. Younger individuals face additional challenges related to career planning, financial hardship and access to age-appropriate services, as do those trying to navigate complex systems such as the National Disability Insurance Scheme (NDIS) or My Aged Care. Public understanding of Parkinson's remains limited, which can lead to stigma-related isolation and delays in seeking help.

What opportunities are available for individuals through advocacy and research?

Advocacy across Australia is growing stronger. Fight Parkinson's is a founding member of the National Parkinson's Alliance, which is leading development of the first National Parkinson's Action Plan—a unified strategy to improve care, research and awareness nationwide. We also engage in ongoing policy reform to embed Parkinson's-informed care across health, aged-care and disability systems. Research is another focus. We fund and support studies that translate scientific discovery into practical solutions, creating tangible improvements in daily life while accelerating progress toward a cure. Our community actively co-designs research projects to ensure they reflect lived experiences and real-world needs.

How else can people with Parkinson's in Australia get involved?

There are a lot of ways to participate: joining or leading a peer-support group, volunteering for events or committees, contributing to research or clinical trials, fundraising and sharing personal stories to raise awareness, for example. Community involvement is central to everything we do. Every contribution—whether through time, advocacy or shared experience—helps move the Parkinson's community closer to a future defined by equity, innovation and hope.

Australia

Dr. Melissa McConaghy, founder of PD Warrior®

Tell us about PD Warrior and its mission.

PD Warrior was created to close a critical gap in Parkinson's care: making exercise a core part of treatment. We offer personalized programs for individuals and training for health professionals. Our flagship program, the 10 Week Challenge, combines tailored exercise and education and reinforces self-efficacy and motivation. It's available online and at licensed facilities globally. Each plan is adapted to a person's goals, symptoms and limitations. Most importantly, it's built to be sustainable. In a recent survey, 94% of participants reported continuing to exercise after completing the program—and that's exactly what we aim for.

Are the priorities for the Parkinson's community in Australia similar to those in other developed nations?

Yes. We're fortunate to have broad access to Parkinson's medications—they're both affordable and widely available. In metropolitan areas, patients also benefit from strong access to neurologists and movement disorder specialists. However, access drops off significantly outside the cities. For rural and remote communities, connecting with local experts or community-based programs remains a major hurdle. Expanding access to resources—especially through virtual programs—is an ongoing priority.

What are the barriers to achieving those priorities?

Geography and infrastructure play a major role. While around 80% of Australia's population lives on the east coast, many people with Parkinson's live in rural or remote areas, where access to specialists and community support programs is limited. Another difference lies in our fragmented support structure. Australia has eight states and territories, each with its own Parkinson's organization. These groups often operate independently, with limited coordination and redundant administrative costs. Unfortunately, that means valuable resources that could go toward community programs or research are sometimes lost in inefficiencies. We also have a federal Parkinson's organization, but it's not well integrated with state-level efforts.

How can the Australian Parkinson's community help the cause?

One of the most exciting changes over the past 15 years is the growing momentum among people with Parkinson's. There's a noticeable shift—people are speaking up, asking more questions and demanding better care. That kind of grassroots advocacy is powerful. There are many ways to contribute: building community, joining support groups or even advocating for better services. The state-based organizations have done a great job of building supportive communities and providing education, wellness programs and opportunities for people to engage meaningfully.

Canada

Scott Townsend, Vice President, Philanthropy, Marketing & Communications, Parkinson Canada

What is Parkinson Canada's mission?

We're driven by the belief that everyone deserves to live a life without limits. Every step we take is guided by our vision of a brighter future, where those living with Parkinson's and their care partners are equipped with the tools, support and hope they need to thrive.

Our mission is to empower and inspire people living with Parkinson's and their care partners to thrive and live courageously. Our vision is a world where no one is limited by Parkinson's.

What are the priorities for the Parkinson's community in Canada?

We're united by a shared commitment to improving quality of life and driving progress. Key areas of focus include advancing research, strengthening access to care, expanding support services and raising public awareness.

Could you tell us a little more about the challenges specific to Canada?

Access to timely, specialized care can be limited—especially in rural and remote areas—and services like physiotherapy and mental health support vary widely across the country.

Many experience financial strain from out-of-pocket costs for medications and care, while care partners often lack formal support. There's also a continued need for greater public awareness, improved coordination of care and sustained investment in research across Canada.

What opportunities are there for Canadians to contribute?

People can volunteer their time, lend their voice to advocacy, participate in fundraising events like SuperWalk or donate to help fund research and support services. Every contribution—whether through time, action or financial support—helps.

Europe

Cathy Molohan, a board member of Parkinson's Europe

What's the central focus of Parkinson's Europe?

Parkinson's Europe serves as the umbrella organization for national Parkinson's organizations across the continent. Its mission is to support member organizations, elevate patient voices and promote best practices across countries. We focus on improving care standards, increasing awareness and strengthening advocacy efforts at both national and EU levels. The organization plays a critical role in unifying fragmented efforts and sharing knowledge across borders to improve outcomes for people with Parkinson's.

What are some of the top challenges facing the Parkinson's community in Europe?

Awareness and access remain two of the biggest challenges, and they vary across Europe. In some countries, Parkinson's simply isn't as well-known as it is in the United States—many people don't even recognize the disease unless it's explained to them. Part of this difference may stem from the high-profile advocates in the U.S., like Michael J. Fox and Muhammad Ali, who brought widespread attention to the condition, and a broader cultural understanding of what it means to be a patient voice. In Europe, advocacy often needs to be explained.

Access to specialists is another issue, particularly movement disorder specialists and Parkinson's nurses. While some countries have relatively good access to neurologists, comprehensive, team-based care is much less common. As a result, many people with Parkinson's go years after diagnosis without receiving guidance on key lifestyle interventions like exercise, speech therapy or nutritional support.

Health systems also differ—Europe offers universal coverage, but access to movement disorder specialists and holistic care can be limited. In Ireland, for example, the ratio of neurologists to the population is among the lowest in Europe. The result is often more fragmented, siloed care.

Can you tell us a little about the state of patient advocacy in Europe?

Advocacy in Europe is still emerging. While there are growing efforts at the grassroots level, there's less infrastructure around patient advocacy compared to the U.S. Individuals often advocate for themselves in navigating care systems, and there's a need for more structured roles in both government and industry collaboration. Research participation is also less visible and harder to access in some regions. More education and outreach are needed to empower people with Parkinson's to get involved and feel that their voices matter.

India

Dr. Maria Barretto, CEO, Parkinson's Disease and Movement Disorder Society (PDMDS)

Tell us about the origins and mission of PDMDS.

The Parkinson's Disease and Movement Disorder Society (PDMDS) was founded in 2001 by Dr. B.S. Singhal, a neurologist, to improve the quality of life for people living with Parkinson's across India. When I joined in 2004, the organization began building community-based care programs to reach those without access to specialized treatment. Its mission is twofold: to serve people with Parkinson's through accessible, evidence-based programs and to raise awareness among healthcare professionals, families and the public. Our goal is to make care available where people live, not simply where hospitals exist.

What are some of the biggest challenges facing the Parkinson's community in India?

With a population of 1.4 billion and only around 5,000 neurologists—who are mostly concentrated in large cities—access to care is the single greatest barrier. Urban centers like Mumbai may offer free rehabilitation programs through public hospitals, but distance, cost, transportation and overcrowding limit availability. In rural and tribal regions, knowledge of Parkinson's is limited and even basic diagnosis is challenging. Parkinson's is sometimes mistaken for aging, leading people to seek help from traditional healers instead of medical professionals. Many live for years without knowing they have the disease, while community health workers often lack training in neurological conditions.

How has PDMDS addressed these gaps in care?

We designed the PDMDS Model of Care, an evidence-based, community-driven program that integrates physiotherapy, speech therapy and psychological support into group sessions. Beginning in Mumbai, it has grown to 70-plus centers nationwide and now reaches more than 8,000 people each month. The model emphasizes practical, low-cost solutions—such as training local health workers and social work students—to adapt care to each region's realities. Dance, music and culturally relevant activities make exercise and social interaction approachable, while technology extends access to virtual sessions across the country. We've learned that therapy doesn't have to be expensive to be effective—it just has to be consistent and local.

What opportunities exist for people in India to get involved?

PDMDS has built a strong peer-driven network where people with Parkinson's act as "ambassadors," sharing their experiences and encouraging participation. The organization collaborates with government agencies and other nonprofits to foster awareness through shared resources. For those newly diagnosed, involvement can begin simply—for instance, joining a local or online support group, volunteering at a community center or helping educate others. We can't wait for perfect conditions: We must work with what we have and turn challenges into opportunities.

Malaysia

*Sara Lew, President, Malaysian Parkinson's
Disease Association*

Can you tell us a bit about the Malaysian Parkinson's Disease Association and its mission?

The Malaysian Parkinson's Disease Association (MPDA) was founded in 1994 by a group of dedicated volunteers to raise awareness, provide education and build a supportive community for people living with Parkinson's. What began as a small gathering of patients and caregivers has grown into a national organization based in Kuala Lumpur, offering regular support group meetings, educational talks and information sessions.

MPDA's mission is centered on education, empowerment and connection to bridge the gap between medical care and the everyday needs of people with Parkinson's and their families. Our goal is simple: to help people live their best lives. We do that by bringing people together with support groups and reminding them that they're not alone. The first step is understanding Parkinson's—learning about it, being informed and staying connected. During the pandemic, we expanded our online programs to reach members nationwide, including many who had never before been able to attend in-person events.

What are some of the challenges facing the Parkinson's community in Malaysia?

Malaysia is a relatively small country, yet access to care varies widely. In Kuala Lumpur, neurologists and movement disorder specialists are available, but in smaller states like East Malaysia, many people must travel long distances to receive care. Awareness also remains a big challenge. In rural areas, few people recognize Parkinson's as a neurological condition, and education about the disease is limited.

Both public and private healthcare systems exist. Public hospitals are often crowded with short appointment times, and private treatment can be costly. On a positive note, our association successfully advocated for Parkinson's disease to be officially recognized as a disability. That's made a significant difference: The government now provides ongoing care for Parkinson's patients, and medications are available free of charge.

What opportunities exist for Malaysians to get involved or make an impact?

Awareness and volunteerism are steadily growing across Malaysia. We're always seeking individuals who are willing to advocate and share their stories. Personal storytelling—whether through public events, social media or simple word-of-mouth—has proven to be a powerful way to educate others and inspire understanding. There are other ways to contribute: volunteering at MPDA events, joining support groups, assisting with outreach and helping raise funds, to name a few. The future lies in collaboration—bringing together people with Parkinson's, health professionals and researchers to build a more connected approach to awareness and care across Malaysia.

New Zealand

Andrew Bell, Chief Executive, Parkinson's New Zealand

Can you share some background on Parkinson's New Zealand?

Parkinson's New Zealand is a nonprofit focused on helping people live positively with Parkinson's. Our mission centers on providing information, education and support, empowering people with Parkinson's and their care partners to take ownership of their condition. We promote self-management strategies and lifestyle interventions like exercise and diet, and we deliver care through a team of nurses, physiotherapists, social workers and other qualified allied health professionals who offer practical, day-to-day advice. Our motto reflects our day-to-day approach: *Living Positively with Parkinson's.*

Tell us about some of the key challenges facing the Parkinson's community in New Zealand.

The biggest challenges here are access to care, underdiagnosis and the uneven distribution of services across the country's small but geographically dispersed population. New Zealand has only 48 neurologists spread across the entire country, servicing about 13,000 people with Parkinson's, so coverage is an issue. And very few doctors specialize in movement disorders.

Most people rely on the public health system (based on the British National Health Service), which often leads to long wait times and minimal access to expert care. Some only see a neurologist once a year. This puts the burden of management back on the individual, making education and self-directed action critical for living well with Parkinson's.

The geography also presents a challenge—New Zealand is a long, narrow country with people spread across rural and urban areas. Most patients see general practitioners, who may have limited Parkinson's experience. As a result, Parkinson's is often underdiagnosed and poorly managed unless the person is proactive in seeking expert care.

How can the country's Parkinson's community help each other?

People with Parkinson's in New Zealand are encouraged to advocate for themselves in the health system and connect with the community. Parkinson's New Zealand employs 20 specialist clinicians to offer education, support and community-based care, but the organization receives no government funding. As a result, people with Parkinson's and care partners are a vital part of the advocacy effort, helping to petition the government for greater support. And we encourage people to form social groups to grab a meal at a pub or see a movie—just connect.

Spain (Catalan)

*Laura Morer, Executive Director, Catalan
Parkinson's Association*

**Tell us about the Catalan Parkinson's Association and its role in
supporting those with the disease.**

The Catalan Parkinson's Association, based in Barcelona, was
founded in 1985 and is Spain's oldest Parkinson's organization.
Its mission is to improve the quality of life of people with the
disease and their families through education, therapy and social
support. It operates seven groups, providing access to physiotherapy, speech therapy, psychological counseling and occupational
therapy. We also work closely with hospitals, neurologists and
rehabilitation centers to drive continuity of care. While we origi-
nally focused on in-person services, we now use online platforms
to reach people in rural areas.

**How would you describe the current state of awareness and
access to care in Catalonia?**

Awareness of Parkinson's has improved, but access remains uneven.
Major cities like Barcelona have specialized units and rehabilitation programs, but in smaller towns, neurologists are scarce and
therapy options limited. Spain's regional public health system
covers neurological consultations, medications and treatments—
including deep brain stimulation—but rehabilitation and ongoing
therapy aren't always included, leaving patients to pay privately
or rely on organizations like ours.

What are some of the challenges and opportunities for advocacy and community support?

Advocacy in Spain is growing, though much of the work is still led by patient associations rather than government institutions. We raise awareness through media campaigns, workshops and collaborations with universities and research centers. We're also working to educate the public in everyday spaces—like supermarkets and schools—so that people with Parkinson's are better understood and accepted. Volunteerism is strong, with family members, caregivers and those living with the disease playing active roles in programs, fundraising and peer mentoring. We encourage people to educate themselves, empowering them to become their own advocates for better treatments and care.

How can people in Spain contribute or get involved?

There are a lot of ways to make a difference. People can volunteer with the Association, join support groups or take part in research projects conducted in partnership with hospitals and universities. We encourage members to become ambassadors—they can share their stories publicly or online to help raise awareness and advocate from a personal perspective. Research participation is another growing opportunity, as hospitals increasingly reach out to us to connect with potential volunteers. It's great to see more researchers providing direct feedback to study participants, helping them see the firsthand role they play and the impact of their involvement. The Catalan Parkinson's Association believes that collective advocacy—patients, families, caregivers and professionals working together—is the key to building a more inclusive and informed future for everyone living with Parkinson's.

United Kingdom

Caroline Rassell, Chief Executive, Parkinson's UK

Juliet Tizzard, Director of External Relations, Parkinson's UK

Could you share some insights about Parkinson's UK and its mission?

Founded in 1969, Parkinson's UK is a national charity that supports 160,000-plus people living with Parkinson's in the UK. It works across the country: partnering with the National Health Service (NHS), funding scientific studies, training health professionals and running local groups that empower individuals to live well. We are people-led, centering the voices of those with lived experience in everything from strategy to storytelling.

What are the key areas of focus for the Parkinson's community in the UK?

Parkinson's UK centers its work around three core pillars: Hope, Control and Care. *Hope* is about accelerating research to find better treatments and a cure. *Control* focuses on helping people live well with Parkinson's by promoting exercise, nutrition, creative expression and peer support. And *Care* advocates for timely, equitable access to specialist nurses, therapists, consultants and neurologists. Parkinson's UK also educates healthcare professionals across the NHS to improve the standard of care.

Tell us a little about some of the current challenges in the UK.

Access to care remains one of the most urgent and widespread issues. In some areas, people can wait more than two years just to receive a diagnosis. Around 20% of people with Parkinson's still don't have access to a specialist nurse. Many emergency hospital visits—which could have been prevented with proper support—remain common.

Access to therapies such as speech, occupational and physiotherapy is inconsistent, leaving many without critical tools to manage their condition. Opportunities to participate in research aren't typically integrated into the healthcare system and government investment in Parkinson's research also remains relatively low.

Are there opportunities for people to contribute?

Parkinson's UK has a strong volunteer base of more than 4,000 individuals and a network of over 450 local branches that not only offer peer support but are becoming community hubs for exercise and social engagement. Anyone can get involved in advocacy efforts at both the local and national level, whether by campaigning to protect essential services or by pushing for better standards of care. We also encourage people with Parkinson's to share their personal stories through videos or written testimonials to raise awareness and influence policy.

Your organization created a Tech Guide for the Parkinson's community a few years ago. How did that come about?

About two years ago, we started getting overwhelmed with requests seeking advice about apps, devices and technology. So, we developed an online Tech Guide where people can share their experiences. We also curate practical information—details on how easy something is to buy, to open, to set up—on our website. We're not grading products, but we are providing a space where the Parkinson's community can weigh in on what's worked for them.

Major Parkinson's Organizations

AMERICAN PARKINSON DISEASE ASSOCIATION (APDA)
www.apdaparkinson.org

BRIAN GRANT FOUNDATION
www.briangrant.org

CATALAN ASSOCIATION FOR PARKINSON'S
www.parkinsoncat.org

CURE PARKINSON'S
www.cureparkinsons.org.uk

DAVIS PHINNEY FOUNDATION
www.davisphinneyfoundation.org

FIGHT PARKINSON'S (AUSTRALIA)
www.fightparkinsons.org.au

INTERNATIONAL PARKINSON AND MOVEMENT DISORDER SOCIETY
www.movementdisorders.org

THE KIRK GIBSON FOUNDATION
www.kirkgibsonfoundation.org

MALAYSIAN PARKINSON'S DISEASE ASSOCIATION
mpda.org.my

THE MICHAEL J. FOX FOUNDATION
www.michaeljfox.org

PARKINSON CANADA
www.parkinson.ca

PARKINSON'S AFRICA
www.parkinsonsafrica.org

PARKINSON'S DISEASE AND MOVEMENT DISORDER SOCIETY (INDIA)
www.parkinsonssocietyindia.com

PARKINSON'S EUROPE
www.parkinsonseurope.org

PARKINSON'S FOUNDATION
www.parkinson.org

PARKINSON'S NEW ZEALAND
www.parkinsons.org.nz

PARKINSON'S UK
www.parkinsons.org.uk

PD AVENGERS
www.pdavengers.com

PD WARRIOR (AUSTRALIA)
www.pdwarrior.com

PMD ALLIANCE
www.pmdalliance.org

WORLD PARKINSON'S COALITION (WPC)
www.worldpdcoalition.org

For the latest list of resources, see the *Living Parkinson's* website, livingparkinsons.com.

REFERENCES

Chapter 1

1. Dorsey ER, Zafar M, Lettenberger SE, Pawlik ME, Kinel D, Frissen M, Schneider RB, Kieburtz K, Tanner CM, De Miranda BR, Goldman SM, Bloem BR. Trichloroethylene: An Invisible Cause of Parkinson's Disease? J Parkinsons Dis. 2023;13(2):203-218.

2. Bandura, A. (1977). *Self-Efficacy: Toward a Unifying Theory of Behavioral Change. Psychological Review*, 84(2), 191–215.

3. Bandura, A. (1997). *Self-Efficacy: The Exercise of Control.* New York: W.H. Freeman.

4. Schunk, D. H., & DiBenedetto, M. K. (2020). Motivation and social cognitive theory. *Contemporary Educational Psychology*, 60, 101832.

5. O'Leary A. Self-efficacy and health. Behav Res Ther. 1985;23(4):437-51.

6. Estrada-Bellmann, Ingrid & Meléndez-Flores, Jesús & Camara-Lemarroy, Carlos & Castillo-Torres, Sergio. (2021). Determinants of self-efficacy in patients with Parkinson's disease. Arquivos de Neuro-Psiquiatria. 79. 686-691.

7. van der Heide A, Meinders MJ, Speckens AEM, Peerbolte TF, Bloem BR, Helmich RC. Stress and Mindfulness in Parkinson's Disease: Clinical Effects and Potential Underlying Mechanisms. Mov Disord. 2021 Jan;36(1):64-70.

Chapter 4

8. Yale School of Medicine. (2024). High-intensity Exercise May Reverse Neurodegeneration in Parkinson's Disease. https://medicine.yale.edu/news-article/high-intensity-exercise-can-reverse-neurodegeneration-in-parkinsons-disease

9. Larson D, Yeh C, Rafferty M, Bega D. High satisfaction and improved quality of life with Rock Steady Boxing in Parkinson's disease: results of a large-scale survey. Disabil Rehabil. 2022 Oct;44(20):6034-6041.

Chapter 5

10. American Parkinson Disease Association (APDA). (2021). The Effects of the MIND and Mediterranean Diets on Parkinson's Disease. https://www.apdaparkinson.org/article/mind-and-mediterranean-diets

11. Hughes KC, Gao X, Kim IY, Wang M, Weisskopf MG, Schwarzschild MA, Ascherio A. Intake of dairy foods and risk of Parkinson disease. Neurology. 2017 Jul 4;89(1):46-52.

12. Neth BJ, Bauer BA, Benarroch EE, Savica R. The Role of Intermittent Fasting in Parkinson's Disease. Front Neurol. 2021 Jun 1;12:682184.

13. American Parkinson Disease Association (APDA). (2024). What Worsens Parkinson's Disease's Motor Symptoms? https://www.apdaparkinson.org/article/what-worsens-parkinsons-disease

14. Yi Q, Yu-Peng C, Jiang-Ting L, Jing-Yi L, Qi-Xiong Q, Dan-Lei W, Jing-Wei Z, Zhi-Juan M, Yong-Jie X, Zhe M and Zheng X (2022) Worse Sleep Quality Aggravates the Motor and Non-Motor Symptoms in Parkinson's Disease. Front. Aging Neurosci. 14:887094.

15. Parkinson's Foundation. (2021). How Stress and Stress Management Impact Parkinson's. https://www.parkinson.org/blog/science-news/stress-management-impact

16. Environmental Working Group. EWG's Shopper's Guide to Pesticides in Produce. https://www.ewg.org/foodnews

17. Dorsey ER, Bloem BR. Parkinson's Disease Is Predominantly an Environmental Disease. J Parkinsons Dis. 2024;14(3):451-465.

18. Buettner, D. (2012). *The Blue Zones: 9 Lessons for Living*

Longer from the People Who've Lived the Longest. National Geographic Society.

19. Trinh J, de Vries NM, Chan P, Dekker MCJ, Helmich RC, Bloem BR. The role of lifestyle interventions in symptom management and disease modification in Parkinson's disease. Lancet Neurol. 2026 Jan;25(1):90-102.

Chapter 7

20. Parkinson's Foundation. (n.d.). Current Findings from PD GENEration. https://www.parkinson.org/advancing-research/our-research/pdgeneration/genetics-behind-pd

ACKNOWLEDGEMENTS

Writing *Living Parkinson's* has been one of the most challenging—and most fulfilling—undertakings of my life. In many ways, it documents my journey so far. I don't yet know where this path will take me in the years ahead, but I hope to share new editions as my story continues to unfold.

There are many people I owe thanks to, beginning with the one who truly set me on this course: business writer, author and friend Charlie Slack. It was Charlie who proposed the idea of taking on this project—it took multiple tries before he convinced me—and he has been absolutely critical in bringing it to life. He has been both a mentor and editorial voice, constantly challenging me to keep refining *Living Parkinson's* and making it the best it can be. Without him, this book simply wouldn't exist.

Sincere thanks also to editor and friend Mike Fox (not *that* Mike Fox), whose sharp eye and insightful feedback were instrumental in refining the text. I really appreciate his guidance, commitment and expertise. I also want to acknowledge Linda VonAncken, who provided legal guidance, Tom Jackson for illustrations and Rob Deal for photographs.

I'm deeply grateful to the family and friends who read the manuscript as it evolved, offering both high-level perspectives and detailed editorial comments. Your insights helped shape *Living Parkinson's* into the book it is today.

I also want to acknowledge those who took the time to read and provide feedback on the entire book: Jackie Madwed, Steve Merrifield, Laura Ryan, Mike Wiesner and particularly Melissa Bray, who reviewed multiple versions of *Living Parkinson's* as it progressed.

To my wife Hillary, thank you for your patience during the

many evenings I was tucked away in my office, researching and writing. Thank you for supporting me when I chose to give up time together to focus on this book. To my kids Melissa, Zack, Matt and Jake, your encouragement has meant the world to me. And to all my family and friends, your steady belief in me kept me moving forward.

A special thanks to everyone who agreed to be interviewed for this book: the researchers, advocates and organizational leaders from around the world who generously shared their time, expertise and personal perspectives. Your contributions not only enriched this book but taught me countless lessons along the way.

Lastly, I want to thank my care team: the doctors and health-care professionals who have helped me manage my Parkinson's in a way that enables me to keep doing the things I love, including writing *Living Parkinson's*. Your skill and dedication make it possible for me to keep showing up in the fight.

To all of you, thank you for helping me tell this story.

I would like to acknowledge the use of AI tools, which assisted me with research and refining some of the language in this book. All ideas, perspectives and personal stories remain my own or those of the individuals and organizations interviewed.

ABOUT THE AUTHOR

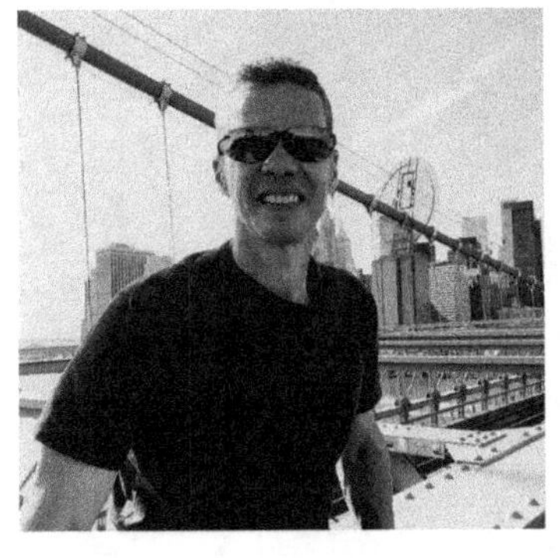

Steve Yellen is a seasoned technology marketing leader whose professional career has spanned pricing strategy, product marketing and executive leadership across a wide range of technology-driven companies. With more than 25 years of experience guiding both startups and global enterprises, Steve has built a reputation for turning complex challenges into transformative results.

An engineer by training, Steve holds a Master of Science in Electrical Engineering from Cornell University and a Master of Business Administration in Marketing from the University of Connecticut.

Diagnosed with Parkinson's in his mid 50s, Steve turned to data, research and personal experimentation to understand and manage the disease. Knowing that exercise is the only potential way to slow progression, he made fitness central to his life, training daily and competing in triathlons and obstacle course races (e.g., Spartans) and even racing up the Empire State Building stairs.

Beyond personal health and wellness, Steve is deeply involved in Parkinson's advocacy and research.

Living Parkinson's shares the strategies and real-life stories that have helped Steve and others live full lives with Parkinson's.

Steve lives in Connecticut and actively promotes the *Living Parkinson's* message at events and online at livingparkinsons.com and on Instagram at @LivingParkinsons. He can be reached directly via the website.